UTERINE FIBROID DIET

FOR WOMEN

A Comprehensive Guide with Nutrient-Packed Recipes for Hormonal Balance and Uterine Wellness to Thrive Naturally

KELLY C. BROWN

Table of Contents

INTRODUCTION

Clara struggled with uterine fibroids, which had a significant influence on her everyday life. Determined to find a natural remedy, she came upon the transformational effect of a Uterine Fibroid Diet for Women. Clara's journey started when she embraced nutrient-dense meals and avoided trigger foods.

Her meals consisted of leafy greens, cruciferous vegetables, and antioxidant-rich fruits. Clara concentrated on nutrients that promote hormonal balance, such as flaxseed and omega-3 fatty acids. With each nutritious food, she strengthened her body to fight fibroid growth.

Regular exercise supplemented her dietary adjustments by increasing blood circulation and decreasing inflammation. Clara found refuge in yoga and embraced stress-management strategies, comprehending the complex relationship between mind and body.

Months passed, and Clara's devotion paid off. Regular check-ups demonstrated a significant improvement in her uterine fibroid.

The Uterine Fibroid Diet for Women became Clara's ally, demonstrating that feeding the body from inside may result in miraculous recovery.

Welcome to this Uterine Fibroid Diet, a comprehensive guide designed to help women manage and alleviate the effects of uterine fibroids. Uterine fibroids, which are non-cancerous growths in the uterus, may cause pain, excessive monthly flow, and influence general health. The Uterine Fibroid Diet for Women is a planned and powerful dietary plan that aims to treat the underlying causes of fibroid development and boost overall health.

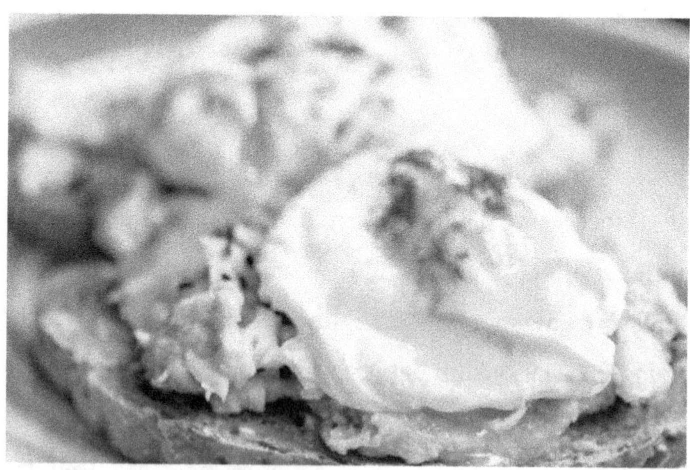

CHAPTER 1: UNDERSTANDING UTERINE FIBROIDS

Uterine fibroids, or leiomyomas, are non-cancerous growths that form in or around the uterus and afflict a large number of people, particularly women of reproductive age. This in-depth look into uterine fibroids attempts to provide light on their sources, symptoms, diagnosis, and possible therapy techniques.

CAUSES AND RISK FACTORS

While the exact causes of uterine fibroids are unknown, genetic, hormonal, and environmental factors are thought to contribute to their development. Hormones including estrogen and progesterone, which play important roles in the menstrual cycle and pregnancy, seem to impact fibroid development. Genetic predisposition, age, and ethnicity all play a role, with African American women being more vulnerable.

SYMPTOMS

Uterine fibroids may cause a range of symptoms, with some people not having any visible consequences.

Common symptoms include:

1. Menstrual Changes: Include heavy bleeding, longer periods, and irregular menstruation.
2. Pelvic discomfort and Pressure: Discomfort or pain in the pelvic area, usually accompanied by a sense of fullness.
3. Frequent Urination: Fibroids pushing on the bladder may cause an increased need to pee.
4. Backache or Leg discomfort: Large fibroids may put pressure on nearby nerves, producing back or leg discomfort.

DIAGNOSIS

Uterine fibroids are normally diagnosed by medical history, pelvic examinations, and imaging investigations.

This may include:

1. Ultrasound: A common and non-invasive approach for visualizing the uterus and detecting fibroids.
2. MRI (Magnetic Resonance Imaging): Produces detailed images that aid in assessing fibroid size and location.

3. Hysteroscopy or Laparoscopy: Hysteroscopy, often known as laparoscopy, is an invasive surgery that allows direct sight of the uterus and is commonly performed for confirmation or in more difficult circumstances.

TYPES OF UTERINE FIBROIDS

Uterine fibroids are classified into many categories based on where they are located in the uterus:

1. Intramural fibroids are located inside the uterine muscle wall.
2. Submucosal fibroids grow into the uterine cavity.
3. Subserosal fibroids grow outward from the uterine wall.
4. Pedunculated fibroids have a stalk that attached them to the uterus.

Understanding the kind and location of fibroids is critical for establishing the best treatment choices.

TREATMENT AND MANAGEMENT

Strategies for uterine fibroids depend on the degree of symptoms, health condition, and reproductive aspirations.

Options include:

1. Watchful Waiting: Monitoring without intervention, appropriate for asymptomatic patients.
2. Medications: Hormonal medicines may help control menstrual periods or minimize bleeding.
3. Minimally Invasive Procedures: Procedures like uterine artery embolization and targeted ultrasound to reduce or remove fibroids.
4. Surgical Interventions: Include hysterectomy or myomectomy in extreme situations.

LIFESTYLE AND DIETARY CONCERNS

According to emerging studies, lifestyle changes such as eating a well-balanced diet, exercising regularly, and managing stress may help relieve symptoms. Specialized recipes that concentrate on nutrition for uterine health are becoming more popular as supplementary methods.

IMPORTANCE OF DIET IN MANAGING FIBROIDS

Maintaining a balanced diet is critical for treating fibroids, which are a prevalent health problem among women. A well-balanced diet promotes general health and may significantly reduce the symptoms and growth of fibroids.

1. Nutrient-Rich Meals: Consuming nutrient-dense meals such as fruits, vegetables, whole grains, and lean meats offers necessary vitamins and minerals. These nutrients aid in the body's natural healing processes and relieve fibroid symptoms.

2. Fiber Intake: A high-fiber diet helps to regulate hormones and promotes regular bowel motions. This may be advantageous for women who have fibroids since hormonal imbalances can lead to their formation and growth.

3. Hydration: Staying hydrated aids in the body's detoxification processes and promotes healthy organ function. Drinking enough of water may help eliminate toxins and promote a healthy balance in the reproductive system.

4. Limiting Processed Foods: Avoiding processed foods, which sometimes include additives and preservatives, may help with fibroid treatment. These additions may disrupt hormonal balance and worsen symptoms.

5. Hormone Balancing: Omega-3 fatty acid-rich meals may help balance hormones and prevent inflammation. Including omega-3-rich foods in your diet, such as fatty fish and flaxseeds, may help you have a healthy hormonal profile.

6. Maintaining a Healthy Weight: Obesity is associated with an increased risk of fibroids and may exacerbate symptoms. A balanced diet and frequent physical exercise may help you control your weight and improve your overall health.

7. Iron-Rich Foods: For women who have excessive monthly flow due to fibroids, eating iron-rich foods is critical for preventing anemia. Leafy greens, lentils, and lean meats are good sources of iron.

8. Mindful Eating: Paying attention to portion sizes and practicing mindful eating may help with weight control and avoid overconsumption of harmful foods.

FOODS TO EAT AND FOODS TO AVOID

FOODS TO EAT

1. Fruits and Vegetables: These foods are high in antioxidants, vitamins, and fiber, which promote general health and may assist with fibroid symptoms. Berries, leafy greens, broccoli, and citrus fruits are great options.

2. Whole Grains: Choose whole grains such as quinoa, brown rice, and oatmeal. They supply important nutrients and help to maintain hormonal balance.

3. Lean Proteins: Include lean protein sources including chicken, fish, tofu, and lentils. Protein promotes tissue healing and helps to maintain muscular mass.

4. Omega-3 Fatty Acids: Include fatty fish such as salmon, chia seeds, and flaxseeds in your daily diet. Omega-3s may aid to decrease inflammation and maintain hormonal balance.

5. Herbs and Spices: Turmeric, ginger, and green tea contain anti-inflammatory qualities that may help women with fibroids. Consider adding these to your meals.

6. Low-Fat Dairy: For a calcium boost without too much saturated fat, look for low-fat dairy products. Yogurt and milk are excellent sources.

7. Iron-Rich Foods: To combat probable anemia caused by excessive monthly flow, consume iron-rich foods such as spinach, lentils, and lean meat.

8. Hydrating Beverages: Drink lots of water to keep hydrated and help the body detoxify naturally. Herbal teas might be an effective option.

FOODS TO LIMIT OR AVOID

1. Red Meat and Processed Meats: High consumption of red and processed meats may lead to inflammation. Limiting these may improve fibroid treatment.

2. High-Fat Meals: Limit your consumption of saturated fats from fried meals, processed snacks, and certain oils. High-fat diets may disrupt hormonal equilibrium.

3. Refined Sugars and Carbohydrates: Limit your intake of sugary snacks, pastries, and refined carbs. These may cause weight gain and may worsen fibroid symptoms.

4. Caffeine and Alcohol: Excessive coffee and alcohol consumption may alter hormonal balance and lead to inflammation. Moderation is crucial.

5. Dairy Products with Added Hormones: To prevent hormonal abnormalities, use hormone-free dairy products.

6. Soy Products: While perspectives on soy differ, some research suggests that excessive soy intake may affect estrogen levels. Consult a healthcare expert for specific guidance.

7. High-Sodium Meals: Limit your consumption of salty meals, since excess salt may lead to water retention and bloating.

8. Non-Organic Produce: When feasible, choose organic fruits and vegetables to reduce your exposure to pesticides, which may disrupt hormone control.

SHOPPING LISTS FOR UTERINE FIBROIDS DIET

Proteins

- Chicken breasts or thighs
- Salmon or other fatty fish
- Tofu or tempeh (for vegetarians/vegans)
- Lentils or chickpeas
- Eggs

Vegetables

- Leafy greens (spinach, kale, collard greens)
- Broccoli
- Brussels sprouts
- Bell peppers
- Avocado

Fruits

- Berries (blueberries, strawberries, raspberries)
- Citrus fruits (oranges, grapefruits)
- Bananas
- Apples
- Kiwi

Whole Grains

- Quinoa
- Brown rice
- Oats
- Whole wheat bread or pasta

Nuts and Seeds

- Chia seeds
- Flaxseeds
- Almonds or walnuts

Dairy or Dairy Alternatives

- Low-fat yogurt
- Milk (cow's milk or plant-based alternatives)
- Cheese (in moderation)

Herbs and Spices

- Turmeric
- Ginger
- Cinnamon
- Garlic
- Fresh herbs (parsley, cilantro, basil)

Beverages

- Water (stay hydrated)
- Herbal teas (chamomile, peppermint, ginger)

Iron-Rich Foods

- Spinach
- Lentils
- Lean meats (chicken, turkey)
- Quinoa

Omega-3 Sources

- Fatty fish (salmon, mackerel)
- Chia seeds
- Flaxseeds
- Walnuts

Low-Fat Dairy

- Low-fat milk or milk alternatives
- Low-fat yogurt

Grains and Legumes

- Whole wheat pasta
- Chickpeas
- Black beans

Sweeteners (in moderation)

- Honey
- Maple syrup

Miscellaneous

- Olive oil (extra virgin)
- Green tea
- Fresh fruits and vegetables for variety and seasonal choices

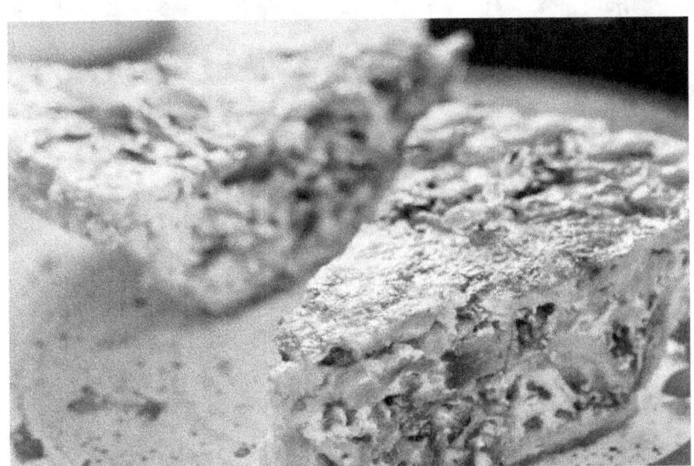

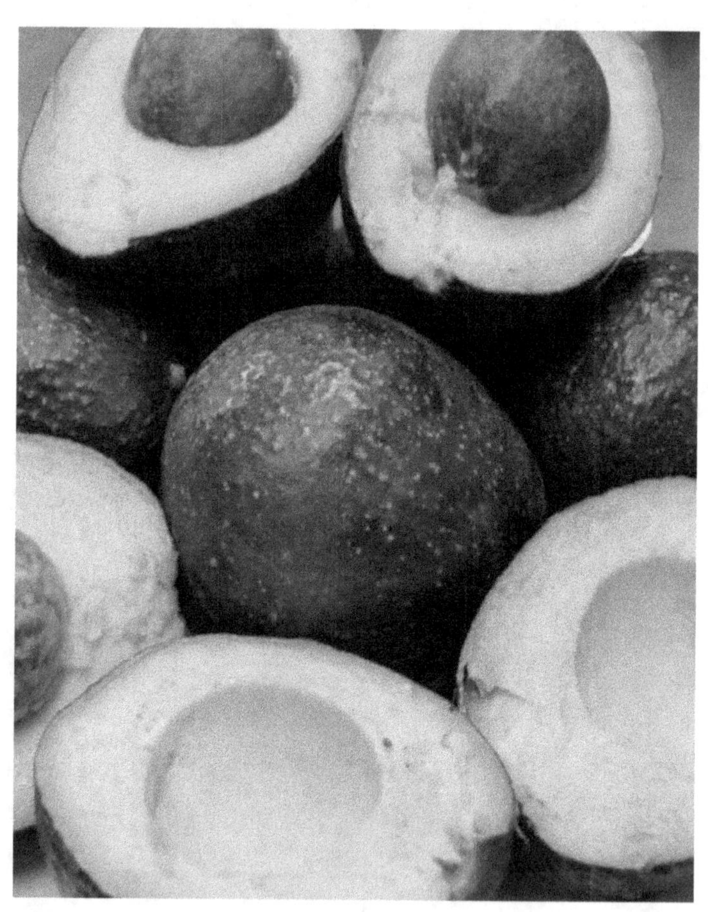

CHAPTER 2: 30-DAY MEAL PLAN

DAY 1

BREAKFAST: Quinoa and Berry Breakfast Bowl

LUNCH: Mediterranean Chickpea Salad Bowl

SNACK: Cucumber Hummus Bites

DINNER: Quinoa and Veggie Stir-Fry

DAY 2

BREAKFAST: Avocado Toast with Poached Egg and Spinach

LUNCH: Vegetable Stir-Fry with Tofu and Brown Rice

SNACK: Apple Slices with Almond Butter

DINNER: Baked Lemon Herb Salmon

DAY 3

BREAKFAST: Fruit and Nut Yogurt Parfait

LUNCH: Caprese Salad with Avocado

SNACK: Yogurt and Berry Parfait Cup

DINNER: Mushroom and Spinach Quiche

DAY 4

BREAKFAST: Spinach and Feta Omelet Wrap

LUNCH: Mango Chickpea Salad Wrap

SNACK: Sliced Avocado with Tomato and Lime

DINNER: Grilled Lemon Garlic Chicken Salad

DAY 5

BREAKFAST: Chia Seed Pudding with Mixed Berries

LUNCH: Lemon Garlic Shrimp and Quinoa Bowl

SNACK: Mango Coconut Chia Pudding

DINNER: Sweet Potato and Chickpea Buddha Bowl

DAY 6

BREAKFAST: Sweet Potato and Black Bean Breakfast Bowl

LUNCH: Grilled Chicken and Vegetable Wrap

SNACK: Nutty Banana Bites

DINNER: One-Pan Lemon Herb Salmon with Roasted Vegetables

DAY 7

BREAKFAST: Cottage Cheese and Pineapple Toast

LUNCH: Quinoa and Black Bean Stuffed Bell Peppers

SNACK: Cottage Cheese and Pineapple Delight

DINNER: Mango Lime Chicken Skewers

DAY 8

BREAKFAST: Banana Nut Overnight Oats

LUNCH: Egg Salad Lettuce Wraps

SNACK: Cherry Almond Energy Bites

DINNER: Vegetarian Quinoa Stuffed Bell Peppers

DAY 9

BREAKFAST: Egg and Veggie Breakfast Wrap

LUNCH: Mango Avocado Chickpea Salad

SNACK: Turmeric Honey Almond Snack

DINNER: Caprese Zucchini Noodles

DAY 10

BREAKFAST: Mango Yogurt Smoothie Bowl

LUNCH: Sesame Ginger Tofu Stir-Fry Bowl

SNACK: Caprese Skewers with Balsamic Glaze

DINNER: Lemon Garlic Shrimp Stir-Fry

DAY 11

BREAKFAST: Apple Cinnamon Overnight Chia Pudding

LUNCH: Sweet Potato and Black Bean Quesadilla

SNACK: Cucumber Hummus Bites

DINNER: Chickpea and Vegetable Curry

DAY 12

BREAKFAST: Peanut Butter Banana Toast

LUNCH: Mediterranean Chickpea and Avocado Salad

SNACK: Apple Slices with Almond Butter

DINNER: Teriyaki Tofu Stir-Fry

DAY 13

BREAKFAST: Turmeric and Blueberry Smoothie

LUNCH: Pesto Zoodles with Cherry Tomatoes and Pine Nuts

SNACK: Yogurt and Berry Parfait Cup

DINNER: Mango Avocado Black Bean Salad

DAY 14

BREAKFAST: Mushroom and Spinach Breakfast Quesadilla

LUNCH: Lemon Herb Shrimp and Quinoa Bowl

SNACK: Mango Coconut Chia Pudding

DINNER: Lemon Garlic Butter Shrimp Pasta

DAY 15

BREAKFAST: Tomato Basil Avocado Toast

LUNCH: Mediterranean Chickpea Salad Bowl

SNACK: Sliced Avocado with Tomato and Lime

DINNER: Mango Lime Chicken Skewers

DAY 16

BREAKFAST: Quinoa and Berry Breakfast Bowl

LUNCH: Mango Basil Chicken Salad

SNACK: Cucumber Hummus Bites

DINNER: Quinoa and Veggie Stir-Fry

DAY 17

BREAKFAST: Avocado Toast with Poached Egg and Spinach

LUNCH: Vegetable Stir-Fry with Tofu and Brown Rice

SNACK: Apple Slices with Almond Butter

DINNER: Baked Lemon Herb Salmon

DAY 18

BREAKFAST: Fruit and Nut Yogurt Parfait

LUNCH: Caprese Salad with Avocado

SNACK: Yogurt and Berry Parfait Cup

DINNER: Mushroom and Spinach Quiche

DAY 19

BREAKFAST: Spinach and Feta Omelette Wrap

LUNCH: Mango Chickpea Salad Wrap

SNACK: Sliced Avocado with Tomato and Lime

DINNER: Grilled Lemon Garlic Chicken Salad

DAY 20

BREAKFAST: Chia Seed Pudding with Mixed Berries

LUNCH: Lemon Garlic Shrimp and Quinoa Bowl

SNACK: Mango Coconut Chia Pudding

DINNER: Sweet Potato and Chickpea Buddha Bowl

DAY 21

BREAKFAST: Sweet Potato and Black Bean Breakfast Bowl

LUNCH: Grilled Chicken and Vegetable Wrap

SNACK: Nutty Banana Bites

DINNER: One-Pan Lemon Herb Salmon with Roasted Vegetables

DAY 22

BREAKFAST: Cottage Cheese and Pineapple Toast
LUNCH: Quinoa and Black Bean Stuffed Bell Peppers
SNACK: Cottage Cheese and Pineapple Delight
DINNER: Mango Lime Chicken Skewers

DAY 23

BREAKFAST: Banana Nut Overnight Oats
LUNCH: Egg Salad Lettuce Wraps
SNACK: Cherry Almond Energy Bites
DINNER: Vegetarian Quinoa Stuffed Bell Peppers

DAY 24

BREAKFAST: Egg and Veggie Breakfast Wrap
LUNCH: Mango Avocado Chickpea Salad
SNACK: Turmeric Honey Almond Snack
DINNER: Caprese Zucchini Noodles

DAY 25

BREAKFAST: Mango Yogurt Smoothie Bowl

LUNCH: Sesame Ginger Tofu Stir-Fry Bowl

SNACK: Caprese Skewers with Balsamic Glaze

DINNER: Lemon Garlic Shrimp Stir-Fry

DAY 26

BREAKFAST: Apple Cinnamon Overnight Chia Pudding

LUNCH: Sweet Potato and Black Bean Quesadilla

SNACK: Cucumber Hummus Bites

DINNER: Chickpea and Vegetable Curry

DAY 27

BREAKFAST: Peanut Butter Banana Toast

LUNCH: Mediterranean Chickpea and Avocado Salad

SNACK: Apple Slices with Almond Butter

DINNER: Teriyaki Tofu Stir-Fry

DAY 28

BREAKFAST: Turmeric and Blueberry Smoothie

LUNCH: Pesto Zoodles with Cherry Tomatoes and Pine Nuts

SNACK: Yogurt and Berry Parfait Cup

DINNER: Mango Avocado Black Bean Salad

DAY 29

BREAKFAST: Mushroom and Spinach Breakfast Quesadilla

LUNCH: Lemon Herb Shrimp and Quinoa Bowl

SNACK: Mango Coconut Chia Pudding

DINNER: Lemon Garlic Butter Shrimp Pasta

DAY 30

BREAKFAST: Tomato Basil Avocado Toast

LUNCH: Mango Basil Chicken Salad

SNACK: Sliced Avocado with Tomato and Lime

DINNER: Teriyaki Tofu Stir-Fry

CHAPTER 3: BREAKFAST DELIGHTS

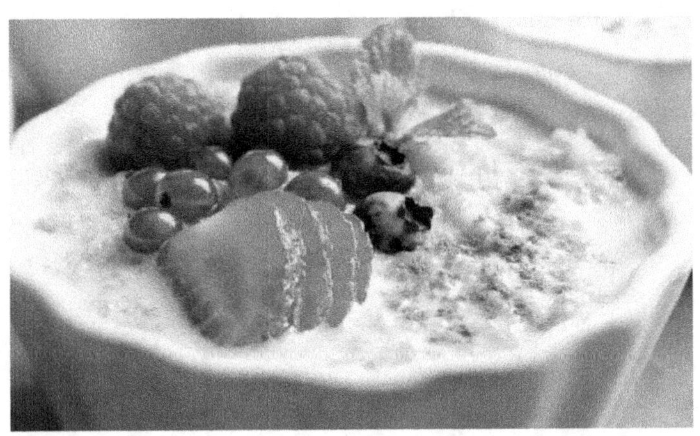

Quinoa and Berry Breakfast Bowl

Ingredients:

- 1 cup cooked quinoa
- 1/2 cup mixed berries (strawberries, blueberries, raspberries)
- 1 tablespoon chia seeds
- 1 tablespoon flaxseeds
- 1/4 cup Greek yogurt
- 1 tablespoon honey or maple syrup
- Handful of nuts (almonds, walnuts, or pistachios)

1. In a bowl, combine the cooked quinoa and mixed berries.
2. Sprinkle chia seeds and flaxseeds over the quinoa and berries mixture.
3. Add a dollop of Greek yogurt on top.
4. Drizzle honey or maple syrup for sweetness.
5. Garnish with a handful of nuts for crunch and extra nutrients.
6. Mix everything together and enjoy this nutrient-packed, fibroid-friendly breakfast!

Avocado Toast with Poached Egg and Spinach

Ingredients:

- 1 slice whole-grain bread
- 1/2 ripe avocado
- 1 large egg
- Handful of fresh spinach
- Salt and pepper to taste
- Optional toppings: red pepper flakes, sliced tomatoes, or a squeeze of lemon

Instructions:

1. Toast the whole-grain bread to your liking.

2. Mash the ripe avocado and spread it evenly on the toasted bread.

3. In a small pan, poach the egg until the whites are set but the yolk is still runny.

4. Place the poached egg on top of the avocado-covered toast.

5. Quickly sauté the fresh spinach in the same pan until wilted, then layer it on the toast.

6. Season with salt and pepper to taste.

7. Optional: Add a sprinkle of red pepper flakes, sliced tomatoes, or a squeeze of lemon for extra flavor.

8. Enjoy this easy and nutritious breakfast that incorporates the goodness of avocado, whole grains, and leafy greens.

Fruit and Nut Yogurt Parfait

Ingredients:
- 1 cup Greek yogurt (unsweetened)
- 1 tablespoon honey or maple syrup
- 1/4 cup granola (choose a low-sugar, whole-grain option)
- 1/2 cup mixed fresh fruits (berries, kiwi, mango, or any preferred fruits)

- 1 tablespoon chopped nuts (almonds, walnuts, or pistachios)

Instructions:

1. In a glass or bowl, layer half of the Greek yogurt.
2. Drizzle half of the honey or maple syrup over the yogurt.
3. Add half of the granola on top of the yogurt layer.
4. Place half of the mixed fresh fruits on the granola.
5. Sprinkle half of the chopped nuts over the fruits.
6. Repeat the layering process with the remaining ingredients.
7. Finish with a final drizzle of honey or maple syrup on top.
8. Grab a spoon and enjoy this delightful and nutritious Fruit and Nut Yogurt Parfait!

Spinach and Feta Omelet Wrap

Ingredients:

- 2 large eggs
- Handful of fresh spinach, chopped
- 2 tablespoons crumbled feta cheese

- Salt and pepper to taste
- 1 whole-grain tortilla

Instructions:

1. Whisk the eggs in a bowl and season with salt and pepper.

2. Heat a non-stick skillet over medium heat and spray with cooking spray.

3. Pour the whisked eggs into the skillet, allowing them to spread evenly.

4. Sprinkle the chopped spinach and crumbled feta evenly over one half of the omelet.

5. Once the edges begin to set, carefully fold the omelet in half using a spatula.

6. Cook for an additional minute until the cheese melts and the omelet is fully cooked.

7. Warm the tortilla in the skillet for about 10 seconds on each side.

8. Slide the omelet onto the tortilla and fold it into a wrap.

Chia Seed Pudding with Mixed Berries

Ingredients:

- 3 tablespoons chia seeds
- 1 cup almond milk (or any preferred milk)

- 1 tablespoon honey or maple syrup
- 1/2 teaspoon vanilla extract
- 1/2 cup mixed berries (strawberries, blueberries, raspberries)

Instructions:

1. In a bowl, combine chia seeds, almond milk, honey or maple syrup, and vanilla extract.
2. Whisk the mixture thoroughly and let it sit for about 5 minutes.
3. Whisk again to break up any clumps of chia seeds, ensuring they are evenly distributed.
4. Cover the bowl and refrigerate overnight or for at least 3-4 hours until it reaches a pudding-like consistency.
5. Before serving, give the chia pudding a good stir.
6. Spoon the chia pudding into a bowl or glass.
7. Top with mixed berries for a burst of freshness and added nutrients.
8. Drizzle a bit more honey or maple syrup if desired.

Sweet Potato and Black Bean Breakfast Bowl

Ingredients:

- 1 medium sweet potato, peeled and diced
- 1/2 cup canned black beans, drained and rinsed
- 1 teaspoon olive oil
- 1/2 teaspoon ground cumin
- 1/4 teaspoon paprika
- Salt and pepper to taste
- 1 large egg
- Fresh cilantro for garnish (optional)

Instructions:

1. In a skillet, heat olive oil over medium heat.
2. Add diced sweet potato to the skillet and cook until tender, about 8-10 minutes.
3. Stir in black beans, ground cumin, paprika, salt, and pepper. Cook for an additional 2-3 minutes until the beans are heated through.
4. In a separate pan, fry the egg to your liking.
5. Spoon the sweet potato and black bean mixture into a bowl.
6. Top with the fried egg.
7. Garnish with fresh cilantro if desired.

Cottage Cheese and Pineapple Toast

Ingredients:

- 1 slice whole-grain bread
- 1/2 cup low-fat cottage cheese
- 1/2 cup fresh pineapple chunks
- 1 tablespoon honey
- A sprinkle of cinnamon (optional)

Instructions:

1. Toast the whole-grain bread to your preference.
2. Spread a generous layer of low-fat cottage cheese over the toasted bread.
3. Arrange fresh pineapple chunks on top of the cottage cheese.
4. Drizzle honey over the pineapple and cottage cheese.
5. Optional: Sprinkle a bit of cinnamon for extra flavor.
6. Enjoy this delightful and quick Cottage Cheese and Pineapple Toast!

Banana Nut Overnight Oats

Ingredients:

- 1/2 cup rolled oats

- 1/2 cup milk (dairy or plant-based)

- 1 ripe banana, mashed

- 1 tablespoon chopped nuts (walnuts, almonds, or pecans)

- 1/2 teaspoon vanilla extract

- 1 teaspoon honey or maple syrup

- A pinch of cinnamon (optional)

Instructions:

1. In a jar or container, combine rolled oats, milk, mashed banana, chopped nuts, vanilla extract, and honey or maple syrup.

2. Mix well and ensure the oats are fully submerged in the liquid.

3. Cover the jar or container and refrigerate overnight.

4. In the morning, give the oats a good stir.

5. Optional: Sprinkle a pinch of cinnamon for extra flavor.

6. Enjoy this quick and nutritious Banana Nut Overnight Oats straight from the refrigerator!

Mango Yogurt Smoothie Bowl

Ingredients:

- 1 cup plain Greek yogurt

- 1/2 cup frozen mango chunks
- 1/2 banana, sliced
- 1 tablespoon chia seeds
- 1 tablespoon shredded coconut
- Handful of granola

Instructions:

1. In a blender, combine Greek yogurt and frozen mango chunks. Blend until smooth.
2. Pour the smoothie into a bowl.
3. Top with banana slices, chia seeds, shredded coconut, and a handful of granola.
4. Customize with additional toppings like nuts or a drizzle of honey if desired.
5. Grab a spoon and enjoy this refreshing Mango Yogurt Smoothie Bowl!

Egg and Veggie Breakfast Wrap

Ingredients:

- 1 whole-grain tortilla
- 2 large eggs, scrambled
- Handful of spinach, chopped
- 1/4 cup cherry tomatoes, halved
- 1/4 cup bell peppers, diced
- Salt and pepper to taste

- Salsa or hot sauce for extra flavor (optional)

Instructions:

1. In a pan, scramble the eggs until cooked to your liking.
2. While eggs are cooking, warm the tortilla in a separate skillet.
3. Spread the scrambled eggs in the center of the tortilla.
4. Top with chopped spinach, cherry tomatoes, and diced bell peppers.
5. Season with salt and pepper.
6. If desired, add a drizzle of salsa or hot sauce for extra flavor.
7. Fold the sides of the tortilla over the egg and veggie mixture.
8. Serve this Egg and Veggie Breakfast Wrap warm and enjoy!

Apple Cinnamon Overnight Chia Pudding

Ingredients:

- 3 tablespoons chia seeds
- 1 cup almond milk (or any preferred milk)
- 1/2 teaspoon ground cinnamon

- 1 small apple, finely chopped
- 1 tablespoon honey or maple syrup
- A handful of sliced almonds (optional)

Instructions:

1. In a bowl, mix chia seeds, almond milk, ground cinnamon, and honey or maple syrup.
2. Stir well to combine, ensuring chia seeds are evenly distributed.
3. Add the finely chopped apple to the mixture and mix again.
4. Cover the bowl and refrigerate overnight.
5. In the morning, give the chia pudding a final stir.
6. Spoon the pudding into a serving dish.
7. Optionally, top with sliced almonds for added crunch.
8. Enjoy this Apple Cinnamon Overnight Chia Pudding, a delightful and easy-to-make breakfast option!

Peanut Butter Banana Toast

Ingredients:

- 1 slice whole-grain bread
- 1 tablespoon peanut butter (unsweetened)
- 1 banana, sliced

- Drizzle of honey (optional)
- Pinch of chia seeds for garnish (optional)

Instructions:

1. Toast the whole-grain bread to your liking.
2. Spread a generous layer of unsweetened peanut butter on the toasted bread.
3. Arrange banana slices over the peanut butter.
4. Optional: Drizzle honey for extra sweetness.
5. If desired, sprinkle a pinch of chia seeds for added texture.
6. Enjoy this quick and satisfying Peanut Butter Banana Toast!

Turmeric and Blueberry Smoothie

Ingredients:

- 1 cup frozen blueberries
- 1/2 banana
- 1 cup almond milk (or any preferred milk)
- 1/2 teaspoon ground turmeric
- 1 tablespoon chia seeds
- 1 tablespoon almond butter
- Optional: a drizzle of honey for sweetness

1. In a blender, combine frozen blueberries, banana, almond milk, ground turmeric, chia seeds, and almond butter.

2. Blend until smooth and creamy.

3. Taste and add a drizzle of honey if additional sweetness is desired.

4. Pour the smoothie into a glass.

5. Enjoy this Turmeric and Blueberry Smoothie, a vibrant and nutrient-rich breakfast option!

Mushroom and Spinach Breakfast Quesadilla

Ingredients:

- 1 whole-grain tortilla
- 1/2 cup sliced mushrooms
- Handful of fresh spinach
- 1/4 cup shredded mozzarella cheese
- 1 teaspoon olive oil
- Salt and pepper to taste
- Salsa or Greek yogurt for dipping (optional)

Instructions:

1. In a pan, sauté sliced mushrooms in olive oil until tender.

2. Add fresh spinach to the pan and cook until wilted.

3. Season with salt and pepper to taste.

4. Place the whole-grain tortilla in the pan and sprinkle shredded mozzarella over half of it.

5. Spoon the sautéed mushrooms and spinach over the cheese.

6. Fold the tortilla in half, covering the filling.

7. Press down with a spatula and cook for a few minutes on each side until the cheese is melted and the tortilla is golden brown.

8. Slice the quesadilla into wedges and serve with salsa or Greek yogurt for dipping.

Tomato Basil Avocado Toast

Ingredients:
- 1 slice whole-grain bread
- 1/2 ripe avocado
- 1 medium tomato, thinly sliced
- Fresh basil leaves
- Olive oil for drizzling
- Salt and pepper to taste

Instructions:
1. Toast the whole-grain bread to your liking.

2. Mash the ripe avocado and spread it evenly on the toasted bread.

3. Arrange thin slices of tomato over the avocado.

4. Place fresh basil leaves on top of the tomato slices.

5. Drizzle olive oil over the toast.

6. Sprinkle with salt and pepper to taste.

7. Enjoy this Tomato Basil Avocado Toast – a simple, fresh, and nutritious breakfast!

Cranberry Almond Yogurt Parfait

Ingredients:

- 1 cup Greek yogurt (unsweetened)
- 1/4 cup dried cranberries
- 2 tablespoons almond slices
- 1 tablespoon honey
- 1/4 teaspoon vanilla extract

Instructions:

1. In a glass or bowl, layer half of the Greek yogurt.

2. Sprinkle half of the dried cranberries and almond slices over the yogurt.

3. Drizzle honey and add a dash of vanilla extract.

4. Repeat the layering process with the remaining ingredients.

5. Finish with a final drizzle of honey on top.

6. Mix everything together and enjoy this Cranberry Almond Yogurt Parfait!

Peach and Mint Smoothie Bowl

Ingredients:

- 1 ripe peach, sliced
- 1/2 banana
- 1/2 cup almond milk (or any preferred milk)
- Handful of fresh mint leaves
- 1 tablespoon chia seeds
- 1 tablespoon unsweetened coconut flakes

Instructions:

1. In a blender, combine ripe peach slices, banana, almond milk, fresh mint leaves, and chia seeds.

2. Blend until smooth and creamy.

3. Pour the smoothie into a bowl.

4. Top with additional peach slices and a sprinkle of unsweetened coconut flakes.

5. Enjoy this Peach and Mint Smoothie Bowl, a refreshing and easy-to-make breakfast option!

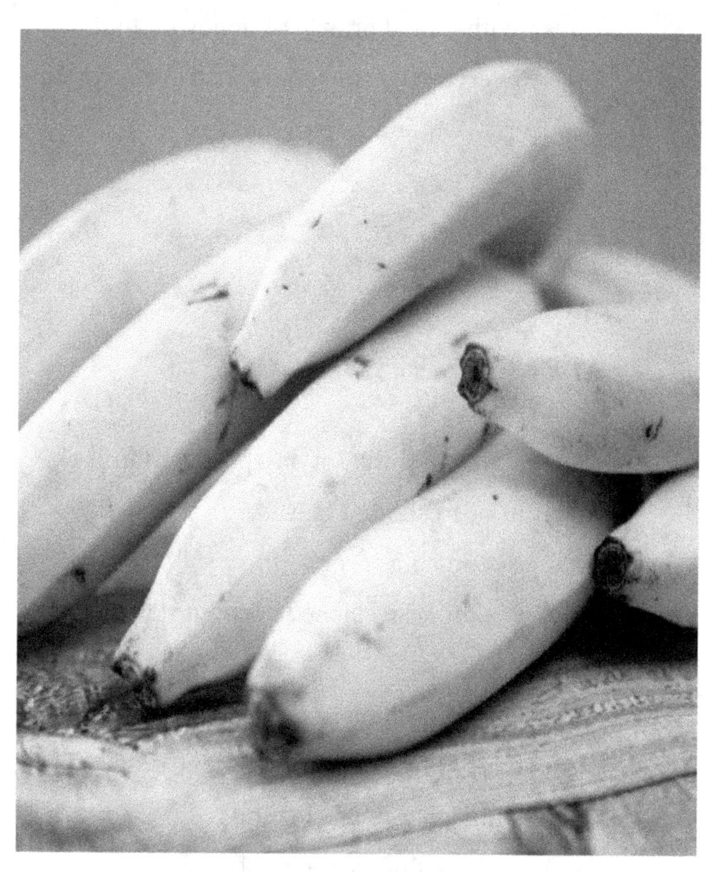

CHAPTER 4: LUNCH FOR HEALING

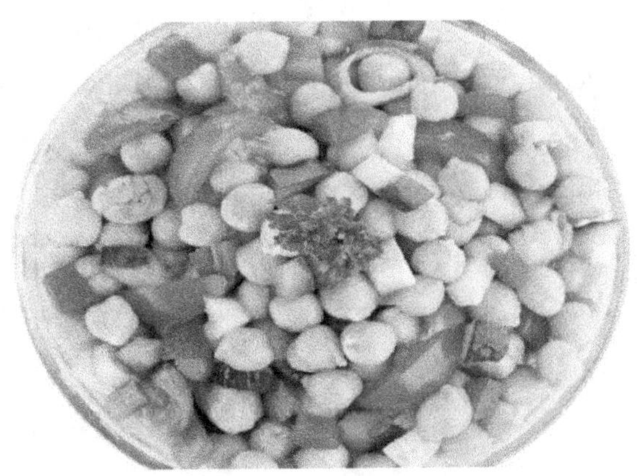

Mediterranean Chickpea Salad Bowl

Ingredients:

- 1 can (15 oz) chickpeas, drained and rinsed
- 1 cup cherry tomatoes, halved
- 1 cucumber, diced
- 1/4 cup red onion, finely chopped
- 1/4 cup Kalamata olives, sliced
- 1/4 cup crumbled feta cheese
- Handful of fresh parsley, chopped

For the Lemon-Herb Dressing:

- 3 tablespoons extra virgin olive oil
- Juice of 1 lemon

- 1 teaspoon dried oregano
- Salt and pepper to taste

Instructions:

1. In a large bowl, combine chickpeas, cherry tomatoes, cucumber, red onion, Kalamata olives, and feta cheese.
2. In a small jar, whisk together olive oil, lemon juice, dried oregano, salt, and pepper to create the dressing.
3. Pour the Lemon-Herb Dressing over the chickpea salad.
4. Toss everything together until well coated.
5. Garnish the salad with fresh parsley.
6. Serve immediately or refrigerate for later.

Vegetable Stir-Fry with Tofu and Brown Rice

Ingredients:

- 1 cup firm tofu, cubed
- 1 cup broccoli florets
- 1 bell pepper, thinly sliced
- 1 carrot, julienned
- 1 cup snap peas, ends trimmed
- 2 tablespoons low-sodium soy sauce

- 1 tablespoon sesame oil
- 1 teaspoon ginger, minced
- 2 cloves garlic, minced
- 1 cup cooked brown rice

Instructions:

1. In a wok or large skillet, heat sesame oil over medium-high heat.
2. Add tofu cubes and stir-fry until golden brown on all sides.
3. Add minced ginger and garlic to the wok, sauté for 30 seconds.
4. Add broccoli, bell pepper, carrot, and snap peas to the wok. Stir-fry for 5-7 minutes until vegetables are tender-crisp.
5. Pour low-sodium soy sauce over the stir-fry and toss everything together.
6. Add the cooked brown rice to the wok and stir to combine.
7. Cook for an additional 2-3 minutes until the rice is heated through.
8. Serve this Vegetable Stir-Fry with Tofu and Brown Rice as a quick and wholesome lunch option.

Caprese Salad with Avocado

Ingredients:

- 2 large tomatoes, sliced
- 1 ripe avocado, sliced
- 1 cup fresh mozzarella balls (or diced mozzarella)
- Fresh basil leaves
- 2 tablespoons balsamic glaze
- 2 tablespoons extra virgin olive oil
- Salt and pepper to taste

Instructions:

1. Arrange tomato slices, avocado slices, and fresh mozzarella on a serving platter.
2. Tuck fresh basil leaves among the tomato and avocado slices.
3. Drizzle balsamic glaze and extra virgin olive oil over the salad.
4. Sprinkle with salt and pepper to taste.
5. Gently toss the salad or serve it as a beautifully layered dish.
6. Enjoy this refreshing Caprese Salad with Avocado as a light and flavorful lunch option.

Mango Chickpea Salad Wrap

Ingredients:

- 1 can (15 oz) chickpeas, drained and rinsed
- 1 ripe mango, diced
- 1/2 red onion, finely chopped
- 1/4 cup fresh cilantro, chopped
- 1 tablespoon lime juice
- 1 teaspoon cumin powder
- Salt and pepper to taste
- Whole-grain wraps or tortillas
- Fresh spinach leaves

Instructions:

1. In a bowl, combine chickpeas, diced mango, red onion, cilantro, lime juice, cumin powder, salt, and pepper.
2. Mash some chickpeas lightly to create a textured mixture.
3. Warm the whole-grain wraps or tortillas.
4. Place a layer of fresh spinach leaves on each wrap.
5. Spoon the mango-chickpea mixture onto the spinach.
6. Fold the sides of the wrap and roll it up.

7. Slice in half if desired, and secure with toothpicks.

8. Serve these Mango Chickpea Salad Wraps as a quick and flavorful lunch option.

Lemon Garlic Shrimp and Quinoa Bowl

Ingredients:

- 1 cup cooked quinoa
- 8 oz shrimp, peeled and deveined
- 2 tablespoons olive oil
- 3 cloves garlic, minced
- Zest of 1 lemon
- Juice of 1 lemon
- 1 teaspoon dried oregano
- Salt and pepper to taste
- Fresh parsley for garnish

Instructions:

1. In a skillet, heat olive oil over medium heat.
2. Add minced garlic and sauté until fragrant.
3. Add shrimp to the skillet, cooking until they turn pink, about 2-3 minutes per side.
4. Sprinkle dried oregano over the shrimp.

5. Add cooked quinoa to the skillet, tossing everything together.

6. Zest a lemon over the mixture and squeeze the lemon juice into the skillet.

7. Season with salt and pepper to taste.

8. Garnish with fresh parsley before serving.

Grilled Chicken and Vegetable Wrap

Ingredients:

- 1 boneless, skinless chicken breast
- 1 tablespoon olive oil
- 1 teaspoon paprika
- 1 teaspoon garlic powder
- Salt and pepper to taste
- Whole-grain wrap or tortilla
- Hummus
- Mixed salad greens
- Cherry tomatoes, halved
- Red bell pepper, thinly sliced
- Cucumber, julienned

Instructions:

1. Preheat a grill or grill pan over medium-high heat.

2. Rub the chicken breast with olive oil, paprika, garlic powder, salt, and pepper.

3. Grill the chicken for 5-7 minutes per side or until fully cooked.

4. Let the chicken rest for a few minutes before slicing it into strips.

5. Warm the whole-grain wrap or tortilla.

6. Spread a layer of hummus over the wrap.

7. Arrange sliced grilled chicken, mixed salad greens, cherry tomatoes, red bell pepper, and julienned cucumber on the wrap.

8. Fold the sides and roll up the wrap.

Quinoa and Black Bean Stuffed Bell Peppers

Ingredients:

- 2 bell peppers, halved and seeds removed
- 1 cup cooked quinoa
- 1 cup black beans, canned and rinsed
- 1 cup corn kernels (fresh or frozen)
- 1 cup diced tomatoes
- 1/2 cup red onion, finely chopped
- 1 teaspoon cumin
- 1/2 teaspoon chili powder

- Salt and pepper to taste
- 1/2 cup shredded cheddar cheese (optional)
- Fresh cilantro for garnish

Instructions:

1. Preheat the oven to 375°F (190°C).
2. In a large bowl, mix cooked quinoa, black beans, corn, diced tomatoes, red onion, cumin, chili powder, salt, and pepper.
3. Stuff each bell pepper half with the quinoa and black bean mixture.
4. If desired, sprinkle shredded cheddar cheese on top of each stuffed pepper.
5. Place the stuffed peppers in a baking dish and cover with foil.
6. Bake in the preheated oven for 25-30 minutes or until the peppers are tender.
7. Garnish with fresh cilantro before serving.

Egg Salad Lettuce Wraps

Ingredients:

- 4 hard-boiled eggs, peeled and chopped
- 2 tablespoons plain Greek yogurt
- 1 tablespoon Dijon mustard
- 2 green onions, finely chopped

- Salt and pepper to taste
- Butter lettuce leaves (or any preferred lettuce)
- Avocado slices for topping (optional)
- Radish slices for garnish (optional)

Instructions:

1. In a bowl, mix chopped hard-boiled eggs, Greek yogurt, Dijon mustard, chopped green onions, salt, and pepper.
2. Spoon the egg salad onto individual lettuce leaves.
3. If desired, top with avocado slices and garnish with radish slices.
4. Wrap the lettuce around the egg salad, creating lettuce wraps.
5. Serve these Egg Salad Lettuce Wraps as a light and satisfying lunch.

Mango Avocado Chickpea Salad

Ingredients:

- 1 can (15 oz) chickpeas, drained and rinsed
- 1 ripe mango, diced
- 1 avocado, diced
- 1/4 cup red onion, finely chopped
- 1/4 cup fresh cilantro, chopped

- Juice of 1 lime
- 2 tablespoons olive oil
- Salt and pepper to taste
- Mixed salad greens

Instructions:

1. In a large bowl, combine chickpeas, diced mango, diced avocado, red onion, and cilantro.
2. In a small bowl, whisk together lime juice, olive oil, salt, and pepper to create the dressing.
3. Pour the dressing over the chickpea salad and toss gently.
4. Serve the Mango Avocado Chickpea Salad over a bed of mixed salad greens.

Sesame Ginger Tofu Stir-Fry Bowl

Ingredients:

- 1 cup firm tofu, cubed
- 2 cups mixed stir-fry vegetables (broccoli, bell peppers, snap peas)
- 1 tablespoon sesame oil
- 2 tablespoons low-sodium soy sauce
- 1 tablespoon rice vinegar
- 1 tablespoon maple syrup or honey
- 1 teaspoon fresh ginger, minced

- 1 clove garlic, minced
- 2 cups cooked brown rice or quinoa

Instructions:

1. In a wok or large skillet, heat sesame oil over medium-high heat.
2. Add cubed tofu and stir-fry until golden brown on all sides.
3. Add minced ginger and garlic, sauté for 30 seconds.
4. Add mixed vegetables to the wok and stir-fry until they are tender-crisp.
5. In a small bowl, mix soy sauce, rice vinegar, and maple syrup or honey.
6. Pour the sauce over the tofu and vegetables, tossing to coat evenly.
7. Serve the Sesame Ginger Tofu Stir-Fry over cooked brown rice or quinoa.

Sweet Potato and Black Bean Quesadilla

Ingredients:

- 1 large sweet potato, peeled and diced
- 1 can (15 oz) black beans, drained and rinsed
- 1 teaspoon cumin

- 1/2 teaspoon smoked paprika
- Salt and pepper to taste
- 4 whole-grain tortillas
- 1 cup shredded cheese (cheddar or Mexican blend)
- Salsa and Greek yogurt for serving

Instructions:

1. Boil or steam the diced sweet potato until tender. Mash it in a bowl.
2. In a separate bowl, mix black beans with cumin, smoked paprika, salt, and pepper.
3. Lay out the tortillas and spread mashed sweet potato on one half of each tortilla.
4. Spoon the seasoned black beans over the sweet potato.
5. Sprinkle shredded cheese over the beans and fold the tortillas in half.
6. In a pan over medium heat, cook the quesadillas for 2-3 minutes on each side until the cheese is melted and tortillas are golden.
7. Slice and serve with salsa and a dollop of Greek yogurt.

Mediterranean Chickpea and Avocado Salad

Ingredients:

- 1 can (15 oz) chickpeas, drained and rinsed
- 1 cucumber, diced
- 1 cup cherry tomatoes, halved
- 1/4 cup red onion, finely chopped
- 1/4 cup Kalamata olives, sliced
- 1 avocado, diced
- Feta cheese crumbles (optional)
- Fresh parsley, chopped

For the Lemon-Oregano Dressing:

- 3 tablespoons extra virgin olive oil
- Juice of 1 lemon
- 1 teaspoon dried oregano
- Salt and pepper to taste

Instructions:

1. In a large bowl, combine chickpeas, diced cucumber, cherry tomatoes, red onion, Kalamata olives, and diced avocado.

2. In a small jar, whisk together olive oil, lemon juice, dried oregano, salt, and pepper to create the dressing.

3. Pour the Lemon-Oregano Dressing over the salad and toss gently to coat.

4. If desired, sprinkle feta cheese crumbles over the salad.

5. Garnish with fresh parsley.

6. Serve immediately and enjoy this refreshing Mediterranean Chickpea and Avocado Salad.

Pesto Zoodles with Cherry Tomatoes and Pine Nuts

Ingredients:

- 2 large zucchini, spiralized into zoodles
- 1 cup cherry tomatoes, halved
- 2 tablespoons pine nuts, toasted
- Fresh basil leaves for garnish

For the Pesto Sauce:

- 2 cups fresh basil leaves
- 1/2 cup grated Parmesan cheese
- 1/3 cup extra virgin olive oil
- 1/4 cup pine nuts
- 2 cloves garlic, minced
- Salt and pepper to taste

Instructions:

1. In a blender or food processor, combine fresh basil, Parmesan cheese, pine nuts, garlic, salt, and pepper.
2. While blending, slowly add the olive oil until the pesto reaches a smooth consistency.
3. In a large pan, sauté zoodles over medium heat for 2-3 minutes until just tender.
4. Add cherry tomatoes to the pan and cook for an additional 1-2 minutes.
5. Toss the zoodles and tomatoes with the prepared pesto sauce until evenly coated.
6. Toast pine nuts in a dry pan over medium heat for 1-2 minutes, stirring frequently.
7. Serve the Pesto Zoodles topped with toasted pine nuts and garnished with fresh basil leaves.

Lemon Herb Shrimp and Quinoa Bowl

Ingredients:

- 1 cup cooked quinoa
- 8 oz shrimp, peeled and deveined
- 1 tablespoon olive oil
- Juice of 1 lemon
- 1 teaspoon dried thyme

- 1 teaspoon dried rosemary
- Salt and pepper to taste
- Mixed greens for serving
- Cherry tomatoes for garnish

Instructions:

1. In a bowl, toss shrimp with olive oil, lemon juice, dried thyme, dried rosemary, salt, and pepper.
2. Heat a skillet over medium-high heat and cook shrimp for 2-3 minutes per side until they are opaque.
3. Arrange a bed of mixed greens on a plate.
4. Spoon cooked quinoa over the greens.
5. Place the lemon herb shrimp on top of the quinoa.
6. Garnish with cherry tomatoes.
7. Serve immediately and enjoy this Lemon Herb Shrimp and Quinoa Bowl.

Mango Basil Chicken Salad

Ingredients:

- 1 cup cooked chicken breast, shredded or diced
- 1 ripe mango, diced
- 1/4 cup red onion, finely chopped

- Fresh basil leaves, torn
- 2 tablespoons lime juice
- 1 tablespoon extra virgin olive oil
- Salt and pepper to taste
- Mixed salad greens or lettuce cups for serving

Instructions:

1. In a bowl, combine cooked chicken, diced mango, chopped red onion, and torn basil leaves.
2. In a small jar, whisk together lime juice, extra virgin olive oil, salt, and pepper to create the dressing.
3. Pour the dressing over the chicken mixture and toss gently to combine.
4. Serve the Mango Basil Chicken Salad over a bed of mixed salad greens or inside lettuce cups.

Chickpea and Veggie Buddha Bowl

Ingredients:

- 1 cup cooked quinoa or brown rice
- 1 can (15 oz) chickpeas, drained and rinsed
- 1 cup cherry tomatoes, halved
- 1 cucumber, diced
- 1/2 red bell pepper, sliced
- 1/4 cup red onion, finely chopped

- Hummus for dressing
- Fresh parsley for garnish

Instructions:

1. Arrange the cooked quinoa or brown rice at the base of a bowl.
2. In sections, add chickpeas, cherry tomatoes, diced cucumber, sliced red bell pepper, and chopped red onion.
3. Drizzle hummus over the bowl as a dressing.
4. Garnish with fresh parsley.
5. Mix the ingredients together just before eating to combine flavors.

Avocado Turkey Wrap

Ingredients:

- 1 whole-grain wrap or tortilla
- 4 oz lean turkey slices
- 1/2 avocado, sliced
- Handful of spinach leaves
- 1 tablespoon Greek yogurt
- 1 teaspoon Dijon mustard
- Salt and pepper to taste

Instructions:

1. Lay out the whole-grain wrap or tortilla on a clean surface.
2. Spread Greek yogurt evenly over the wrap.
3. Place a layer of spinach leaves on one side of the wrap.
4. Arrange turkey slices and avocado slices over the spinach.
5. Drizzle Dijon mustard over the ingredients.
6. Sprinkle with salt and pepper to taste.
7. Fold the sides of the wrap and roll it up.
8. Slice in half if desired.

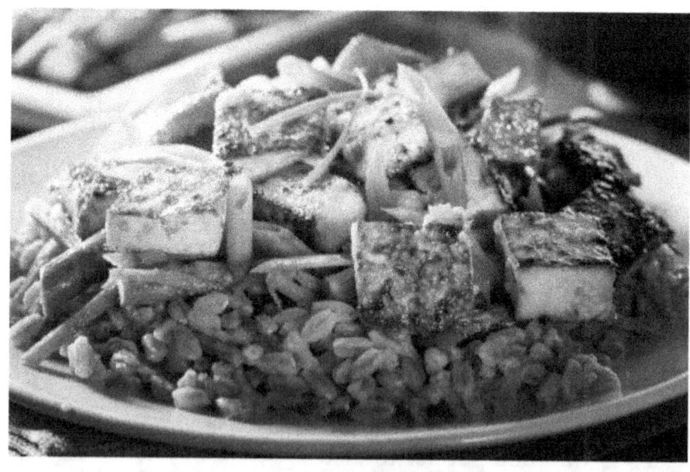

CHAPTER 5: SNACK AND DESSERT OPTIONS

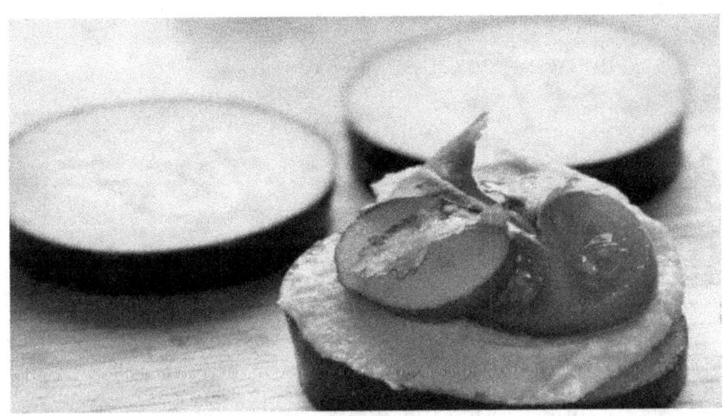

Cucumber Hummus Bites

Ingredients:

- 1 cucumber, sliced into rounds
- 1/2 cup hummus (homemade or store-bought)
- Cherry tomatoes, halved
- Fresh parsley or dill for garnish

Instructions:

1. Slice the cucumber into rounds, creating a base for the bites.
2. Place a small dollop of hummus on each cucumber round.
3. Top with a halved cherry tomato.

4. Garnish with fresh parsley or dill.

5. Arrange the Cucumber Hummus Bites on a
    serving plate.

6. Serve and enjoy this quick, refreshing, and
    nutrient-packed snack!

Apple Slices with Almond Butter

Ingredients:

- 1 apple, cored and sliced
- 2 tablespoons almond butter (unsweetened)
- 1 tablespoon chia seeds (optional)
- Cinnamon for sprinkling

Instructions:

1. Core and slice the apple into wedges.

2. Spread almond butter on each apple slice.

3. If desired, sprinkle chia seeds for an extra
    nutritional boost.

4. Lightly dust with cinnamon for added flavor.

5. Arrange the Apple Slices with Almond Butter on
    a plate.

6. Enjoy this simple yet satisfying snack that
    combines the natural sweetness of apples with
    the richness of almond butter.

Yogurt and Berry Parfait Cup

Ingredients:

- 1/2 cup Greek yogurt (unsweetened)
- 1/4 cup mixed berries (strawberries, blueberries, raspberries)
- 1 tablespoon granola (unsweetened)
- Drizzle of honey or maple syrup (optional)
- Mint leaves for garnish (optional)

Instructions:

1. In a cup or small bowl, layer half of the Greek yogurt.
2. Add a layer of mixed berries on top of the yogurt.
3. Sprinkle granola over the berries.
4. Repeat the layering process with the remaining ingredients.
5. If desired, drizzle honey or maple syrup for sweetness.
6. Garnish with mint leaves for a fresh touch.
7. Serve this Yogurt and Berry Parfait Cup as a quick, delightful, and nutrient-packed snack!

Mango Coconut Chia Pudding

Ingredients:

- 1/4 cup chia seeds
- 1 cup coconut milk (unsweetened)
- 1 ripe mango, diced
- Shredded coconut for topping (optional)

Instructions:

1. In a bowl or jar, mix chia seeds and coconut milk.
2. Stir well and let it sit for a few minutes.
3. Stir again to ensure chia seeds are evenly distributed.
4. Cover and refrigerate for at least 2 hours or overnight.
5. Before serving, give it a final stir.
6. Top with diced mango.
7. Optional: Sprinkle shredded coconut for added texture.
8. Enjoy this Mango Coconut Chia Pudding as a quick, tropical-inspired snack!

Sliced Avocado with Tomato and Lime

Ingredients:

- 1 ripe avocado, sliced
- 1 medium-sized tomato, sliced
- Fresh lime wedges
- Sprinkle of sea salt
- Optional: Red pepper flakes for a kick

Instructions:

1. Arrange avocado slices on a plate.
2. Place tomato slices on top of the avocado.
3. Squeeze fresh lime juice over the avocado and tomato.
4. Sprinkle with a pinch of sea salt.
5. Optional: Add red pepper flakes for a hint of spice.
6. Serve and enjoy this simple, nutrient-rich snack that combines the creaminess of avocado with the freshness of tomatoes.

Nutty Banana Bites

Ingredients:

- 1 banana, peeled and sliced
- 2 tablespoons almond butter (unsweetened)

- 1 tablespoon chopped nuts (walnuts, almonds, or your choice)
- Optional: Drizzle of honey

Instructions:

1. Slice the banana into bite-sized pieces.
2. Spread a small amount of almond butter on each banana slice.
3. Sprinkle chopped nuts over the almond butter.
4. Optional: Drizzle with honey for added sweetness.
5. Arrange the Nutty Banana Bites on a plate or tray.
6. Enjoy this quick and satisfying snack!

Cottage Cheese and Pineapple Delight

Ingredients:

- 1/2 cup low-fat cottage cheese
- 1/2 cup fresh pineapple chunks
- 1 tablespoon shredded coconut (unsweetened)
- Optional: A sprinkle of cinnamon

Instructions:

1. In a bowl, scoop low-fat cottage cheese.
2. Add fresh pineapple chunks to the cottage cheese.

3. Sprinkle shredded coconut over the mixture.

4. Optional: Add a sprinkle of cinnamon for extra flavor.

5. Gently mix the ingredients.

6. Enjoy this Cottage Cheese and Pineapple Delight as a quick, protein-rich, and refreshing snack!

Cherry Almond Energy Bites

Ingredients:

- 1 cup dried cherries
- 1 cup almonds
- 1 tablespoon chia seeds
- 1 tablespoon honey
- Shredded coconut for rolling (optional)

Instructions:

1. In a food processor, combine dried cherries, almonds, chia seeds, and honey.

2. Pulse until the mixture reaches a dough-like consistency.

3. Scoop out small portions and roll them into bite-sized balls.

4. Optional: Roll the energy bites in shredded coconut for extra texture.

5. Place the Cherry Almond Energy Bites on a plate.

6. Refrigerate for at least 30 minutes before serving.

7. Enjoy these delicious and nutritious bites as a quick snack!

Turmeric Honey Almond Snack

Ingredients:
- 1 cup raw almonds
- 1 tablespoon honey
- 1/2 teaspoon ground turmeric
- Pinch of black pepper (to enhance turmeric absorption)

Instructions:

1. In a bowl, combine raw almonds, honey, ground turmeric, and a pinch of black pepper.

2. Toss the almonds until they are evenly coated.

3. Spread the almonds on a baking sheet lined with parchment paper.

4. Bake in a preheated oven at 350°F (180°C) for about 10 minutes or until lightly toasted.

5. Allow the almonds to cool completely before serving.

6. Enjoy these Turmeric Honey Almonds as a flavorful and anti-inflammatory snack!

Caprese Skewers with Balsamic Glaze

Ingredients:

- Cherry tomatoes
- Fresh mozzarella balls
- Fresh basil leaves
- Balsamic glaze

Instructions:

1. Take a toothpick or small skewer.
2. Thread one cherry tomato, one fresh mozzarella ball, and one fresh basil leaf onto each skewer.
3. Repeat for as many skewers as desired.
4. Arrange the Caprese Skewers on a serving plate.
5. Drizzle with balsamic glaze just before serving.
6. Enjoy these flavorful and easy-to-make Caprese Skewers as a light and satisfying snack.

Mango Salsa with Cucumber Slices

Ingredients:

- 1 ripe mango, diced
- 1/4 cup red onion, finely chopped

- 1/4 cup cilantro, chopped
- 1 jalapeño, seeded and minced
- Juice of 1 lime
- Pinch of salt
- Cucumber slices for serving

Instructions:

1. In a bowl, combine diced mango, red onion, cilantro, jalapeño, lime juice, and a pinch of salt.
2. Mix well to ensure even distribution of flavors.
3. Refrigerate for at least 15 minutes to let the flavors meld.
4. Serve the Mango Salsa with Cucumber Slices for a refreshing and low-calorie snack.
5. Enjoy the vibrant combination of sweet and savory flavors in this easy-to-make snack!

Chia Seed Berry Pudding

Ingredients:

- 3 tablespoons chia seeds
- 1 cup almond milk (unsweetened)
- 1 teaspoon vanilla extract
- Mixed berries (strawberries, blueberries, raspberries)
- Drizzle of honey or maple syrup (optional)

Instructions:

1. In a bowl or jar, mix chia seeds, almond milk, and vanilla extract.
2. Stir well and let it sit for a few minutes.
3. Stir again to ensure chia seeds are evenly distributed.
4. Cover and refrigerate for at least 2 hours or overnight.
5. Before serving, give it a final stir.
6. Top with mixed berries.
7. Optional: Drizzle with honey or maple syrup for added sweetness.
8. Enjoy this Chia Seed Berry Pudding as a simple, nutritious, and delightful dessert.

Frozen Banana Bites

Ingredients:

- 2 bananas, peeled and sliced into rounds
- 2 tablespoons dark chocolate, melted
- 1 tablespoon unsweetened shredded coconut
- Chopped nuts (almonds, walnuts) for topping

Instructions:

1. Line a tray with parchment paper.

2. Dip each banana slice into the melted dark chocolate, coating it partially.

3. Place the chocolate-coated banana slices on the prepared tray.

4. Sprinkle shredded coconut over the chocolate-coated part of each banana slice.

5. Top with chopped nuts.

6. Place the tray in the freezer for at least 1 hour or until the chocolate hardens.

7. Once frozen, remove and enjoy these delicious Frozen Banana Bites as a sweet and healthy dessert.

Yogurt Parfait with Dark Chocolate and Berries

Ingredients:

- 1 cup Greek yogurt (unsweetened)
- 1 tablespoon dark chocolate chips or chunks
- Mixed berries (strawberries, blueberries, raspberries)
- Drizzle of honey or maple syrup (optional)

Instructions:

1. In a glass or bowl, layer Greek yogurt.

2. Sprinkle dark chocolate chips or chunks over the yogurt.

3. Add a layer of mixed berries on top of the chocolate.

4. Repeat the layering process until you reach the top of the glass or bowl.

5. Optional: Drizzle with honey or maple syrup for sweetness.

6. Serve immediately and enjoy this quick and indulgent Yogurt Parfait with Dark Chocolate and Berries for a delightful dessert.

Apple Cinnamon Baked Oatmeal Cups

Ingredients:

- 1 cup rolled oats
- 1/2 teaspoon baking powder
- 1 teaspoon ground cinnamon
- 1/4 teaspoon salt
- 1/2 cup unsweetened applesauce
- 1/2 cup almond milk (unsweetened)
- 1 tablespoon maple syrup or honey
- 1 medium-sized apple, diced
- Chopped nuts (walnuts or almonds) for topping

Instructions:

1. Preheat your oven to 350°F (180°C) and grease a muffin tin.

2. In a bowl, combine rolled oats, baking powder, ground cinnamon, and salt.

3. Add applesauce, almond milk, maple syrup, and diced apple to the dry ingredients. Mix well.

4. Spoon the mixture into the muffin tin, filling each cup to the top.

5. Top each oatmeal cup with chopped nuts.

6. Bake for 20-25 minutes or until the tops are golden brown.

7. Allow the baked oatmeal cups to cool slightly before serving.

8. Enjoy these Apple Cinnamon Baked Oatmeal Cups as a wholesome and easy dessert option.

No-Bake Berry Cheesecake Parfait

Ingredients:

- 1 cup low-fat cream cheese
- 1 tablespoon honey or maple syrup
- 1 teaspoon vanilla extract
- Mixed berries (strawberries, blueberries, raspberries)

- Granola for topping (optional)

Instructions:

1. In a bowl, whisk together low-fat cream cheese, honey or maple syrup, and vanilla extract until smooth.

2. In serving glasses or bowls, layer the cream cheese mixture and mixed berries.

3. Repeat the layering until you reach the top.

4. Top with granola for added texture if desired.

5. Chill in the refrigerator for at least 30 minutes before serving.

6. Enjoy this No-Bake Berry Cheesecake Parfait as a quick and luscious dessert.

Pineapple Mint Sorbet

Ingredients:

- 2 cups fresh pineapple chunks
- 1/4 cup fresh mint leaves
- 1 tablespoon lime juice
- 2 tablespoons honey or agave syrup

Instructions:

1. Place pineapple chunks, mint leaves, lime juice, and honey in a blender.

2. Blend until smooth.

3. Pour the mixture into a shallow dish and spread it evenly.

4. Freeze for at least 3-4 hours or until the sorbet is firm.

5. Before serving, let the sorbet sit at room temperature for a few minutes to soften slightly.

6. Scoop into bowls or cones.

7. Garnish with a mint sprig if desired.

8. Enjoy this refreshing Pineapple Mint Sorbet as a simple and satisfying dessert.

Dark Chocolate Dipped Strawberries

Ingredients:

- Fresh strawberries, washed and dried
- Dark chocolate chips or chunks (70% cocoa or higher)
- Optional toppings: Chopped nuts, shredded coconut, or sea salt

Instructions:

1. In a microwave-safe bowl, melt the dark chocolate in 30-second intervals, stirring in between until smooth.

2. Hold each strawberry by the green stem and dip it into the melted chocolate, ensuring even coverage.

3. Allow excess chocolate to drip off.

4. Place the dipped strawberries on a parchment-lined tray.

5. If desired, sprinkle chopped nuts, shredded coconut, or a pinch of sea salt over the chocolate-covered part.

6. Let them cool and harden in the refrigerator for at lcast 20 minutes.

7. Enjoy these Dark Chocolate Dipped Strawberries as a delightful and effortless dessert.

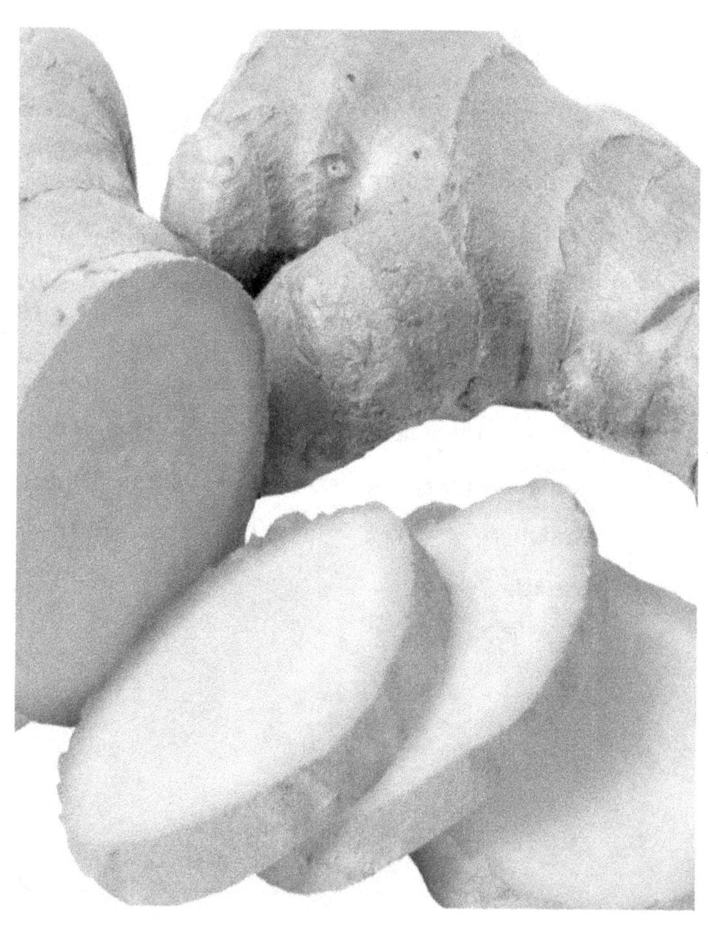

CHAPTER 6: DINNER DELICACIES

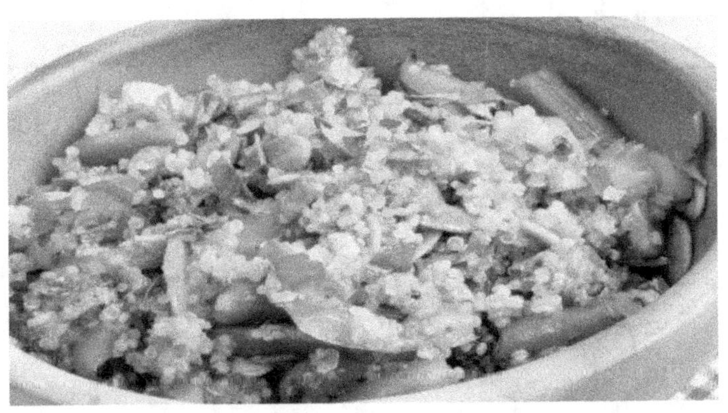

Quinoa and Veggie Stir-Fry

Ingredients:

- 1 cup quinoa, rinsed
- 2 cups water
- 1 tablespoon olive oil
- 1 onion, sliced
- 2 bell peppers (different colors), sliced
- 1 zucchini, sliced
- 1 cup broccoli florets
- 2 cloves garlic, minced
- 1 teaspoon ginger, grated
- 2 tablespoons low-sodium soy sauce

- 1 tablespoon sesame oil
- Sesame seeds for garnish (optional)
- Fresh cilantro for garnish (optional)

Instructions:

1. In a saucepan, combine quinoa and water. Bring to a boil, then reduce heat, cover, and simmer for 15 minutes or until water is absorbed.
2. While quinoa cooks, heat olive oil in a large skillet or wok over medium-high heat.
3. Add sliced onion, bell peppers, zucchini, and broccoli to the skillet. Stir-fry for 5-7 minutes or until vegetables are tender-crisp.
4. Add minced garlic and grated ginger to the vegetables, stir for an additional 1-2 minutes.
5. In a small bowl, mix soy sauce and sesame oil.
6. Add cooked quinoa and the soy sauce mixture to the skillet, tossing everything together until well combined.
7. Cook for an additional 2-3 minutes to heat through.
8. Garnish with sesame seeds and fresh cilantro if desired.
9. Serve this Quinoa and Veggie Stir-Fry as a delicious and nutrient-packed dinner.

Baked Lemon Herb Salmon

Ingredients:

- 2 salmon filets
- 1 lemon, thinly sliced
- 2 tablespoons olive oil
- 1 teaspoon dried oregano
- 1 teaspoon dried thyme
- Salt and pepper to taste
- Fresh parsley for garnish

Instructions:

1. Preheat the oven to 400°F (200°C).
2. Place salmon filets on a baking sheet lined with parchment paper.
3. Drizzle olive oil over each filet and rub to coat.
4. Sprinkle dried oregano, dried thyme, salt, and pepper evenly over the filets.
5. Arrange lemon slices on top of the salmon.
6. Bake in the preheated oven for 15-20 minutes or until the salmon is cooked through and flakes easily with a fork.
7. Garnish with fresh parsley before serving.
8. Enjoy this Baked Lemon Herb Salmon as a simple, flavorful, and healthy dinner option.

Mushroom and Spinach Quiche

Ingredients:

- 1 refrigerated pie crust
- 1 tablespoon olive oil
- 1 onion, finely chopped
- 2 cups mushrooms, sliced
- 2 cups fresh spinach, chopped
- 4 large eggs
- 1 cup milk (dairy or plant-based)
- Salt and pepper to taste
- 1 cup shredded cheese (cheddar, mozzarella, or your choice)

Instructions:

1. Preheat the oven to 375°F (190°C).
2. Press the pie crust into a pie dish, following the package instructions.
3. In a skillet, heat olive oil over medium heat. Add chopped onion and sauté until translucent.
4. Add sliced mushrooms to the skillet and cook until they release their moisture.
5. Add chopped spinach and cook until wilted. Remove from heat.
6. In a bowl, whisk together eggs, milk, salt, and pepper.

7. Spread the mushroom and spinach mixture over the pie crust in the dish.

8. Pour the egg mixture evenly over the veggies.

9. Sprinkle shredded cheese on top.

10. Bake in the preheated oven for 30-35 minutes or until the center is set and the top is golden brown.

11. Allow it to cool for a few minutes before slicing.

12. Serve this Mushroom and Spinach Quiche as a delicious and easy-to-make dinner.

Grilled Lemon Garlic Chicken Salad

Ingredients:

- 2 boneless, skinless chicken breasts
- Zest and juice of 1 lemon
- 3 cloves garlic, minced
- 2 tablespoons olive oil
- Salt and pepper to taste
- Mixed salad greens (lettuce, spinach, arugula)
- Cherry tomatoes, halved
- Cucumber, sliced
- Red onion, thinly sliced
- Feta cheese, crumbled
- Balsamic vinaigrette dressing

Instructions:

1. Preheat the grill or grill pan over medium-high heat.
2. In a bowl, mix lemon zest, lemon juice, minced garlic, olive oil, salt, and pepper.
3. Coat the chicken breasts with the lemon-garlic marinade.
4. Grill the chicken for 6-8 minutes per side or until fully cooked.
5. While the chicken is grilling, prepare the salad by combining mixed greens, cherry tomatoes, cucumber, red onion, and crumbled feta in a large bowl.
6. Once cooked, slice the grilled chicken into strips.
7. Add the sliced chicken to the salad.
8. Drizzle with balsamic vinaigrette dressing and toss to combine.
9. Serve this Grilled Lemon Garlic Chicken Salad as a light, refreshing, and satisfying dinner.

Sweet Potato and Chickpea Buddha Bowl

Ingredients:

- 2 medium-sized sweet potatoes, cubed
- 1 can chickpeas, drained and rinsed
- 2 tablespoons olive oil
- 1 teaspoon cumin
- 1 teaspoon smoked paprika
- Salt and pepper to taste
- Quinoa, cooked according to package instructions
- Avocado, sliced
- Fresh cilantro, chopped
- Tahini dressing (mix 2 tablespoons tahini, 1 tablespoon lemon juice, 1 clove minced garlic, salt, and water to desired consistency)

Instructions:

1. Preheat the oven to 400°F (200°C).
2. In a bowl, toss sweet potato cubes and chickpeas with olive oil, cumin, smoked paprika, salt, and pepper.
3. Spread the sweet potato and chickpea mixture on a baking sheet in a single layer.

4. Roast in the preheated oven for 25-30 minutes or until golden and cooked through, stirring halfway.

5. While roasting, prepare quinoa according to package instructions.

6. Assemble the Buddha bowl by placing quinoa at the base, topping with roasted sweet potatoes and chickpeas, sliced avocado, and chopped cilantro.

7. Drizzle with tahini dressing before serving.

8. Enjoy this Sweet Potato and Chickpea Buddha Bowl as a nutrient-packed and easy-to-make dinner.

One-Pan Lemon Herb Salmon with Roasted Vegetables

Ingredients:

- 2 salmon filets
- 1 pound baby potatoes, halved
- 1 cup baby carrots
- 1 cup cherry tomatoes
- 2 tablespoons olive oil
- Zest and juice of 1 lemon

- 2 teaspoons dried Italian herbs (rosemary, thyme, oregano)
- Salt and pepper to taste
- Fresh parsley for garnish

Instructions:

1. Preheat the oven to 400°F (200°C).
2. Place halved baby potatoes, baby carrots, and cherry tomatoes on a baking sheet.
3. Drizzle with olive oil, lemon zest, lemon juice, dried Italian herbs, salt, and pepper. Toss to coat.
4. Push the vegetables to the sides of the baking sheet, creating space for the salmon filets in the center.
5. Place the salmon filets on the baking sheet, skin side down.
6. Drizzle the salmon with a little olive oil, lemon juice, and sprinkle with salt and pepper.
7. Bake in the preheated oven for 15-20 minutes or until the salmon is cooked through and flakes easily.
8. Garnish with fresh parsley before serving.
9. Enjoy this One-Pan Lemon Herb Salmon with Roasted Vegetables for a delicious and hassle-free dinner.

Mango Lime Chicken Skewers

Ingredients:

- 2 boneless, skinless chicken breasts, cut into cubes
- 1 ripe mango, peeled and diced
- Zest and juice of 1 lime
- 2 tablespoons olive oil
- 1 teaspoon ground cumin
- 1 teaspoon smoked paprika
- Salt and pepper to taste
- Wooden skewers, soaked in water
- Fresh cilantro for garnish

Instructions:

1. In a bowl, combine olive oil, lime zest, lime juice, ground cumin, smoked paprika, salt, and pepper.
2. Add chicken cubes to the marinade, ensuring they are well coated. Let it marinate for at least 15 minutes.
3. Preheat the grill or grill pan over medium-high heat.
4. Thread marinated chicken cubes and diced mango onto the soaked skewers alternately.

5. Grill the skewers for 8-10 minutes, turning occasionally, until the chicken is fully cooked.

6. Garnish with fresh cilantro before serving.

7. Serve these Mango Lime Chicken Skewers with a side salad or rice for a quick and delightful dinner.

Vegetarian Quinoa Stuffed Bell Peppers

Ingredients:

- 4 bell peppers, halved and seeds removed
- 1 cup quinoa, cooked
- 1 can black beans, drained and rinsed
- 1 cup corn kernels (fresh or frozen)
- 1 cup cherry tomatoes, halved
- 1/2 cup red onion, finely chopped
- 1 teaspoon ground cumin
- 1 teaspoon chili powder
- Salt and pepper to taste
- 1 cup shredded cheese (cheddar, Monterey Jack)
- Fresh cilantro for garnish

Instructions:

1. Preheat the oven to 375°F (190°C).

2. In a large bowl, mix cooked quinoa, black beans, corn, cherry tomatoes, red onion, ground cumin, chili powder, salt, and pepper.

3. Spoon the quinoa mixture into the halved bell peppers, pressing down gently.

4. Place the stuffed bell peppers on a baking sheet.

5. Sprinkle shredded cheese on top of each stuffed pepper.

6. Bake in the preheated oven for 20-25 minutes or until the peppers are tender and the cheese is melted and bubbly.

7. Garnish with fresh cilantro before serving.

8. Enjoy these Vegetarian Quinoa Stuffed Bell Peppers as a flavorful and easy-to-make dinner.

Caprese Zucchini Noodles

Ingredients:

- 4 medium zucchinis, spiralized
- 1 cup cherry tomatoes, halved
- 1 cup fresh mozzarella balls
- 1/4 cup fresh basil leaves, torn
- 2 tablespoons extra virgin olive oil
- Balsamic glaze for drizzling
- Salt and pepper to taste

Instructions:

1. Spiralize the zucchinis to create zucchini noodles.
2. In a large bowl, combine zucchini noodles, cherry tomatoes, fresh mozzarella balls, and torn basil leaves.
3. Drizzle extra virgin olive oil over the mixture.
4. Toss the ingredients until well combined.
5. Season with salt and pepper to taste.
6. Divide into serving bowls.
7. Drizzle balsamic glaze over each bowl for added flavor.
8. Enjoy these refreshing Caprese Zucchini Noodles as a light and easy dinner.

Lemon Garlic Shrimp Stir-Fry

Ingredients:

- 1 pound shrimp, peeled and deveined
- 2 tablespoons olive oil
- 3 cloves garlic, minced
- Zest and juice of 1 lemon
- 1 teaspoon red pepper flakes (optional)
- 1 cup snap peas, trimmed
- 1 red bell pepper, thinly sliced

- 2 cups broccoli florets
- Salt and pepper to taste
- Cooked brown rice or cauliflower rice for serving

Instructions:

1. In a large skillet or wok, heat olive oil over medium-high heat.
2. Add minced garlic and red pepper flakes (if using), sauté for about 1 minute until fragrant.
3. Add shrimp to the skillet and cook until they turn pink and opaque.
4. Stir in lemon zest and juice, ensuring the shrimp are well coated.
5. Add snap peas, sliced red bell pepper, and broccoli florets to the skillet. Stir-fry for an additional 3-5 minutes until the vegetables are crisp-tender.
6. Season with salt and pepper to taste.
7. Serve the lemon garlic shrimp and vegetables over cooked brown rice or cauliflower rice.
8. Enjoy this quick and flavorful Lemon Garlic Shrimp Stir-Fry for a delightful dinner.

Chickpea and Vegetable Curry

Ingredients:

- 1 can chickpeas, drained and rinsed
- 1 tablespoon olive oil
- 1 onion, finely chopped
- 2 cloves garlic, minced
- 1 tablespoon curry powder
- 1 teaspoon ground cumin
- 1 teaspoon ground coriander
- 1 teaspoon turmeric
- 1 can diced tomatoes
- 1 cup coconut milk
- 2 cups mixed vegetables (e.g., bell peppers, carrots, peas)
- Salt and pepper to taste
- Fresh cilantro for garnish
- Cooked basmati rice for serving

Instructions:

1. In a large skillet, heat olive oil over medium heat.
2. Add chopped onion and sauté until translucent.
3. Add minced garlic, curry powder, ground cumin, ground coriander, and turmeric. Stir for 1-2 minutes until fragrant.

4. Pour in the diced tomatoes and coconut milk. Bring to a simmer.

5. Add chickpeas and mixed vegetables to the skillet. Stir well.

6. Simmer for 15-20 minutes, allowing the flavors to meld and the vegetables to cook through.

7. Season with salt and pepper to taste.

8. Serve the chickpea and vegetable curry over cooked basmati rice.

9. Garnish with fresh cilantro before serving.

10. Enjoy this easy and flavorful Chickpea and Vegetable Curry for a delicious dinner.

Teriyaki Tofu Stir-Fry

Ingredients:

- 1 block firm tofu, pressed and cubed
- 2 tablespoons soy sauce
- 2 tablespoons teriyaki sauce
- 1 tablespoon sesame oil
- 1 tablespoon olive oil
- 1 bell pepper, thinly sliced
- 1 cup broccoli florets
- 1 carrot, julienned
- 2 cloves garlic, minced

- 1 teaspoon grated ginger
- Green onions for garnish
- Sesame seeds for garnish
- Cooked brown rice for serving

Instructions:

1. In a bowl, mix cubed tofu with soy sauce and teriyaki sauce. Allow it to marinate for 10-15 minutes.
2. Heat olive oil and sesame oil in a large skillet or wok over medium-high heat.
3. Add marinated tofu to the skillet, reserving the marinade. Cook until the tofu is golden brown on all sides.
4. Push the tofu to one side of the skillet and add sliced bell pepper, broccoli florets, julienned carrot, minced garlic, and grated ginger.
5. Stir-fry the vegetables for 3-5 minutes until they are tender-crisp.
6. Pour the reserved marinade over the tofu and vegetables. Stir well to combine.
7. Serve the teriyaki tofu and vegetable stir-fry over cooked brown rice.
8. Garnish with sliced green onions and sesame seeds.

9. Enjoy this Teriyaki Tofu Stir-Fry as a quick, flavorful, and plant-based dinner.

Mango Avocado Black Bean Salad

Ingredients:

- 1 can black beans, drained and rinsed
- 1 ripe mango, peeled and diced
- 1 avocado, diced
- 1 cup cherry tomatoes, halved
- 1/4 cup red onion, finely chopped
- 1/4 cup fresh cilantro, chopped
- Juice of 1 lime
- 2 tablespoons extra virgin olive oil
- Salt and pepper to taste
- Mixed salad greens for serving

Instructions:

1. In a large bowl, combine black beans, diced mango, diced avocado, cherry tomatoes, red onion, and chopped cilantro.
2. In a small bowl, whisk together lime juice, extra virgin olive oil, salt, and pepper.
3. Pour the dressing over the salad and toss gently to coat.

4. Serve the mango avocado black bean salad over a bed of mixed salad greens.

5. Enjoy this refreshing and nutrient-packed salad as a quick and easy dinner.

Lemon Garlic Butter Shrimp Pasta

Ingredients:

- 8 oz linguine or your favorite pasta
- 1 pound large shrimp, peeled and deveined
- 3 tablespoons unsalted butter
- 3 cloves garlic, minced
- Zest and juice of 1 lemon
- Red pepper flakes (optional)
- Salt and black pepper to taste
- Fresh parsley, chopped
- Grated Parmesan cheese for serving

Instructions:

1. Cook the pasta according to package instructions. Drain and set aside.

2. In a large skillet, melt butter over medium heat.

3. Add minced garlic and sauté for about 1 minute until fragrant.

4. Add the shrimp to the skillet, cook for 2-3 minutes on each side until they turn pink and opaque.

5. Stir in lemon zest, lemon juice, red pepper flakes (if using), salt, and black pepper. Cook for an additional 2 minutes.

6. Toss the cooked pasta into the skillet, ensuring it's coated in the flavorful lemon garlic butter sauce.

7. Sprinkle with fresh chopped parsley.

8. Serve the Lemon Garlic Butter Shrimp Pasta with a sprinkle of grated Parmesan cheese.

9. Enjoy this quick and delicious shrimp pasta for a delightful dinner.

CHAPTER 7: SALADS

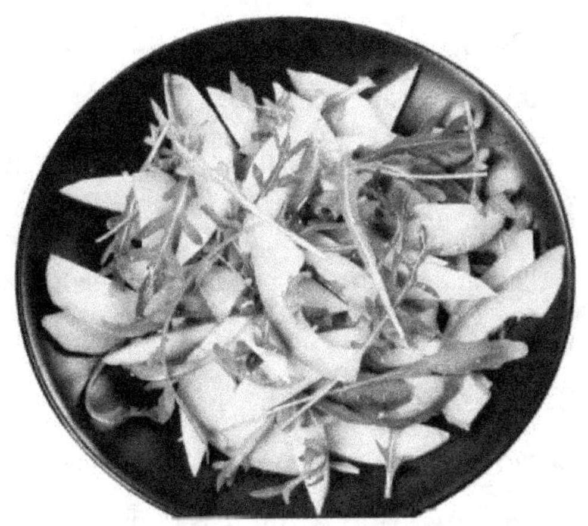

Mango Avocado Arugula Salad

Ingredients:

- 4 cups arugula, washed and dried
- 1 ripe mango, peeled and diced
- 1 avocado, sliced
- 1/4 cup red onion, thinly sliced
- 1/4 cup crumbled goat cheese
- 2 tablespoons extra virgin olive oil
- Juice of 1 lime
- Salt and pepper to taste

Instructions:

1. In a large bowl, combine arugula, diced mango, sliced avocado, thinly sliced red onion, and crumbled goat cheese.
2. In a small bowl, whisk together extra virgin olive oil and lime juice.
3. Drizzle the dressing over the salad and toss gently until well combined.
4. Season with salt and pepper to taste.
5. Serve immediately and enjoy this refreshing Mango Avocado Arugula Salad.

Strawberry Spinach Salad with Balsamic Vinaigrette

Ingredients:

- 4 cups baby spinach, washed and dried
- 1 cup fresh strawberries, hulled and sliced
- 1/4 cup sliced almonds
- 1/4 cup feta cheese, crumbled
- Balsamic Vinaigrette:
    - 3 tablespoons balsamic vinegar
    - 2 tablespoons extra virgin olive oil
    - 1 teaspoon Dijon mustard
    - 1 teaspoon honey

o   Salt and pepper to taste

Instructions:

1. In a large bowl, combine baby spinach, sliced strawberries, sliced almonds, and crumbled feta cheese.

2. In a small bowl, whisk together balsamic vinegar, extra virgin olive oil, Dijon mustard, honey, salt, and pepper to create the vinaigrette.

3. Drizzle the balsamic vinaigrette over the salad and toss gently until ingredients are well coated.

4. Serve immediately and enjoy your vibrant and flavorful Strawberry Spinach Salad.

Cucumber and Tomato Greek Salad

Ingredients:

- 2 cucumbers, diced
- 1 cup cherry tomatoes, halved
- 1/2 cup Kalamata olives, sliced
- 1/4 cup red onion, finely chopped
- 1/2 cup feta cheese, crumbled
- 2 tablespoons extra virgin olive oil
- Juice of 1 lemon
- 1 teaspoon dried oregano
- Salt and pepper to taste

Instructions:

1. In a large bowl, combine diced cucumbers, halved cherry tomatoes, sliced Kalamata olives, finely chopped red onion, and crumbled feta cheese.

2. In a small bowl, whisk together extra virgin olive oil, lemon juice, dried oregano, salt, and pepper.

3. Pour the dressing over the salad and toss gently until all ingredients are well coated.

4. Serve immediately, and enjoy this simple and delicious Cucumber and Tomato Greek Salad.

Apple Walnut Spinach Salad

Ingredients:

- 4 cups baby spinach, washed and dried
- 1 apple, thinly sliced
- 1/2 cup walnuts, roughly chopped
- 1/4 cup dried cranberries
- Feta or goat cheese crumbles (optional)
- Honey Dijon Dressing:
    - 3 tablespoons extra virgin olive oil
    - 1 tablespoon apple cider vinegar
    - 1 tablespoon Dijon mustard

- o   1 tablespoon honey
- o   Salt and pepper to taste

Instructions:

1. In a large bowl, combine baby spinach, thinly sliced apple, chopped walnuts, dried cranberries, and cheese crumbles if desired.
2. In a small bowl, whisk together extra virgin olive oil, apple cider vinegar, Dijon mustard, honey, salt, and pepper to create the dressing.
3. Drizzle the Honey Dijon Dressing over the salad and toss gently until everything is well coated.
4. Serve immediately for a delightful Apple Walnut Spinach Salad.

Caprese Chickpea Salad

Ingredients:

- 1 can chickpeas, drained and rinsed
- 1 cup cherry tomatoes, halved
- 1 cup fresh mozzarella balls
- Fresh basil leaves, torn
- 2 tablespoons extra virgin olive oil
- Balsamic glaze for drizzling
- Salt and pepper to taste

Instructions:

1. In a bowl, combine chickpeas, cherry tomatoes, fresh mozzarella balls, and torn basil leaves.
2. Drizzle extra virgin olive oil over the mixture.
3. Season with salt and pepper to taste.
4. Toss the ingredients until well combined.
5. Drizzle balsamic glaze over the salad just before serving.
6. Serve and enjoy your Caprese Chickpea Salad.

Summer Berry Spinach Salad

Ingredients:

- 4 cups baby spinach, washed and dried
- 1 cup strawberries, sliced
- 1/2 cup blueberries
- 1/2 cup raspberries
- 1/4 cup sliced almonds
- Feta cheese crumbles (optional)
- Poppy Seed Dressing:
    - 3 tablespoons olive oil
    - 2 tablespoons balsamic vinegar
    - 1 tablespoon honey
    - 1 teaspoon poppy seeds
    - Salt and pepper to taste

Instructions:

1. In a large bowl, combine baby spinach, sliced strawberries, blueberries, raspberries, sliced almonds, and feta cheese crumbles if desired.

2. In a small bowl, whisk together olive oil, balsamic vinegar, honey, poppy seeds, salt, and pepper to create the dressing.

3. Drizzle the Poppy Seed Dressing over the salad and toss gently until everything is well coated.

4. Serve immediately and enjoy your refreshing and nutritious Summer Berry Spinach Salad.

Mediterranean Quinoa Salad

Ingredients:

- 1 cup cooked quinoa, cooled
- 1 cucumber, diced
- 1 cup cherry tomatoes, halved
- 1/2 cup Kalamata olives, sliced
- 1/4 cup red onion, finely chopped
- Feta cheese crumbles
- Fresh parsley, chopped

Lemon Herb Dressing:

- 3 tablespoons extra virgin olive oil
- Juice of 1 lemon

- 1 teaspoon dried oregano
- Salt and pepper to taste

Instructions:

1. In a large bowl, combine cooked quinoa, diced cucumber, cherry tomatoes, sliced Kalamata olives, red onion, feta cheese crumbles, and fresh chopped parsley.

2. In a small bowl, whisk together extra virgin olive oil, lemon juice, dried oregano, salt, and pepper to create the dressing.

3. Drizzle the Lemon Herb Dressing over the salad and toss gently until all ingredients are well coated.

4. Serve immediately and enjoy your flavorful Mediterranean Quinoa Salad.

Asian Sesame Noodle Salad

Ingredients:

- 8 oz soba noodles, cooked and cooled
- 1 red bell pepper, thinly sliced
- 1 cup shredded carrots
- 1 cup snap peas, sliced
- 1/4 cup green onions, chopped
- Sesame seeds for garnish

Sesame Soy Dressing:

- 3 tablespoons soy sauce
- 2 tablespoons sesame oil
- 1 tablespoon rice vinegar
- 1 tablespoon honey
- 1 teaspoon grated ginger
- 1 clove garlic, minced

Instructions:

1. In a large bowl, combine cooked and cooled soba noodles, thinly sliced red bell pepper, shredded carrots, sliced snap peas, and chopped green onions.

2. In a small bowl, whisk together soy sauce, sesame oil, rice vinegar, honey, grated ginger, and minced garlic to create the dressing.

3. Pour the Sesame Soy Dressing over the salad and toss gently until all ingredients are well coated.

4. Garnish with sesame seeds.

5. Serve this Asian Sesame Noodle Salad and enjoy!

Avocado Chickpea Salad

Ingredients:

- 1 can chickpeas, drained and rinsed
- 1 avocado, diced
- 1 cup cherry tomatoes, halved
- 1/4 cup red onion, finely chopped
- Fresh cilantro, chopped
- Lime wedges for serving

Lime Vinaigrette:

- 3 tablespoons extra virgin olive oil
- Juice of 2 limes
- 1 teaspoon honey
- Salt and pepper to taste

Instructions:

1. In a bowl, combine chickpeas, diced avocado, cherry tomatoes, red onion, and chopped cilantro.
2. In a small bowl, whisk together extra virgin olive oil, lime juice, honey, salt, and pepper to create the vinaigrette.
3. Drizzle the Lime Vinaigrette over the salad and toss gently until all ingredients are well coated.
4. Serve with lime wedges and enjoy your easy and flavorful Avocado Chickpea Salad.

Peach and Mozzarella Salad

Ingredients:

- 2 ripe peaches, sliced
- 1 cup fresh mozzarella balls
- Handful of arugula
- 1/4 cup basil leaves, torn
- Balsamic glaze for drizzling
- Salt and pepper to taste

Instructions:

1. Arrange sliced peaches, fresh mozzarella balls, and arugula on a serving platter.
2. Sprinkle torn basil leaves over the top.
3. Season with salt and pepper to taste.
4. Drizzle balsamic glaze generously over the salad.
5. Serve this Peach and Mozzarella Salad and enjoy!

Broccoli and Cranberry Slaw

Ingredients:

- 2 cups broccoli slaw mix
- 1/2 cup dried cranberries
- 1/4 cup sunflower seeds

- 1/4 cup Greek yogurt
- 2 tablespoons mayonnaise
- 1 tablespoon apple cider vinegar
- 1 tablespoon honey
- Salt and pepper to taste

Instructions:

1. In a large bowl, combine broccoli slaw mix, dried cranberries, and sunflower seeds.

2. In a small bowl, whisk together Greek yogurt, mayonnaise, apple cider vinegar, honey, salt, and pepper to create the dressing.

3. Pour the dressing over the slaw mixture and toss until well coated.

4. Chill in the refrigerator for at least 30 minutes before serving.

5. Enjoy this quick and easy Broccoli and Cranberry Slaw.

CHAPTER 8: NOURISHING SOUPS AND STEWS

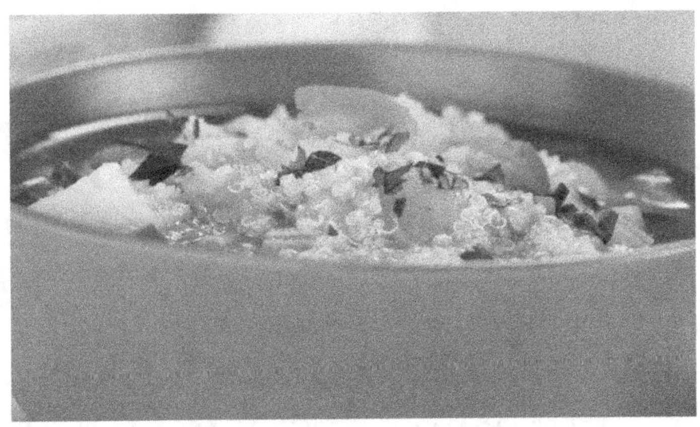

Vegetable Quinoa Soup

Ingredients:

- 1 cup quinoa, rinsed and drained
- 1 onion, finely chopped
- 2 carrots, sliced
- 2 celery stalks, chopped
- 3 cloves garlic, minced
- 1 zucchini, diced
- 1 can (15 oz) diced tomatoes
- 6 cups vegetable broth
- 1 teaspoon dried thyme

- 1 teaspoon dried rosemary
- Salt and pepper to taste
- Fresh parsley for garnish

Instructions:

1. In a large pot, sauté the chopped onion, carrots, and celery over medium heat until softened.
2. Add minced garlic and cook for an additional minute until fragrant.
3. Stir in diced zucchini, diced tomatoes (with their juices), quinoa, vegetable broth, dried thyme, dried rosemary, salt, and pepper.
4. Bring the soup to a boil, then reduce the heat to low, cover, and simmer for 15-20 minutes or until the quinoa is cooked.
5. Adjust seasoning if needed and serve hot.
6. Garnish with fresh parsley before serving.
7. Enjoy this nourishing Vegetable Quinoa Soup.

Lentil and Spinach Stew

Ingredients:

- 1 cup dried lentils, rinsed and drained
- 1 onion, finely chopped
- 2 carrots, diced
- 2 cloves garlic, minced

- 1 teaspoon ground cumin
- 1 teaspoon ground coriander
- 1/2 teaspoon smoked paprika
- 4 cups vegetable broth
- 1 can (14 oz) diced tomatoes
- 3 cups fresh spinach, chopped
- Salt and pepper to taste
- Olive oil for sautéing

Instructions:

1. In a large pot, sauté the chopped onion and diced carrots in olive oil over medium heat until softened.
2. Add minced garlic and sauté for an additional minute until fragrant.
3. Stir in ground cumin, ground coriander, and smoked paprika, coating the vegetables.
4. Add dried lentils, vegetable broth, and diced tomatoes (with their juices) to the pot.
5. Bring the stew to a boil, then reduce the heat to low, cover, and simmer for 25-30 minutes or until lentils are tender.
6. Stir in fresh chopped spinach and cook for an additional 5 minutes until wilted.
7. Season with salt and pepper to taste.

8. Serve hot and enjoy this simple and nutritious Lentil and Spinach Stew.

Tomato Basil Chickpea Soup

Ingredients:

- 1 can (15 oz) chickpeas, drained and rinsed
- 1 onion, finely chopped
- 3 cloves garlic, minced
- 1 can (28 oz) crushed tomatoes
- 4 cups vegetable broth
- 1 teaspoon dried basil
- 1/2 teaspoon dried oregano
- Salt and pepper to taste
- Olive oil for sautéing
- Fresh basil leaves for garnish

Instructions:

1. In a pot, sauté the chopped onion in olive oil over medium heat until translucent.
2. Add minced garlic and cook for an additional minute until fragrant.
3. Pour in the crushed tomatoes, vegetable broth, dried basil, and dried oregano.
4. Add chickpeas to the pot and stir to combine.

5. Bring the soup to a simmer, then reduce the heat to low, cover, and let it cook for 15-20 minutes.

6. Season with salt and pepper to taste.

7. Ladle the soup into bowls and garnish with fresh basil leaves.

8. Serve this Tomato Basil Chickpea Soup and enjoy!

Sweet Potato and Black Bean Chili

Ingredients:

- 2 sweet potatoes, peeled and diced
- 1 can (15 oz) black beans, drained and rinsed
- 1 onion, chopped
- 2 cloves garlic, minced
- 1 can (14 oz) diced tomatoes
- 3 cups vegetable broth
- 1 tablespoon chili powder
- 1 teaspoon ground cumin
- Salt and pepper to taste
- Olive oil for sautéing
- Fresh cilantro for garnish

Instructions:

1. In a large pot, sauté the chopped onion in olive oil over medium heat until softened.

2. Add minced garlic and cook for an additional minute until fragrant.

3. Add diced sweet potatoes, black beans, diced tomatoes (with their juices), vegetable broth, chili powder, and ground cumin to the pot.

4. Bring the chili to a boil, then reduce the heat to low, cover, and simmer for 20-25 minutes or until sweet potatoes are tender.

5. Season with salt and pepper to taste.

6. Ladle the chili into bowls and garnish with fresh cilantro.

7. Enjoy this Sweet Potato and Black Bean Chili as a hearty and easy-to-make option.

Coconut Curry Lentil Soup

Ingredients:
- 1 cup dried red lentils, rinsed and drained
- 1 onion, finely chopped
- 2 carrots, diced
- 3 cloves garlic, minced
- 1 can (14 oz) coconut milk
- 4 cups vegetable broth
- 1 tablespoon curry powder
- 1 teaspoon ground turmeric

- Salt and pepper to taste
- Olive oil for sautéing
- Fresh cilantro for garnish

Instructions:

1. In a pot, sauté the chopped onion in olive oil over medium heat until translucent.
2. Add minced garlic and cook for an additional minute until fragrant.
3. Stir in diced carrots and cook for a few minutes until they begin to soften.
4. Add dried red lentils, coconut milk, vegetable broth, curry powder, and ground turmeric to the pot.
5. Bring the soup to a boil, then reduce the heat to low, cover, and simmer for 15-20 minutes or until lentils are tender.
6. Season with salt and pepper to taste.
7. Ladle the soup into bowls and garnish with fresh cilantro.
8. Serve this Coconut Curry Lentil Soup and enjoy.

Spinach and White Bean Soup

Ingredients:

- 1 can (15 oz) white beans, drained and rinsed

- 4 cups vegetable broth
- 1 onion, finely chopped
- 3 cloves garlic, minced
- 2 cups fresh spinach
- 1 teaspoon dried thyme
- 1/2 teaspoon smoked paprika
- Salt and pepper to taste
- Olive oil for sautéing
- Lemon wedges for serving

Instructions:

1. In a pot, sauté the chopped onion in olive oil over medium heat until translucent.
2. Add minced garlic and cook for an additional minute until fragrant.
3. Pour in vegetable broth, add white beans, dried thyme, and smoked paprika.
4. Bring the soup to a simmer, then reduce the heat to low, cover, and let it cook for 10-15 minutes.
5. Stir in fresh spinach and cook for an additional 5 minutes until wilted.
6. Season with salt and pepper to taste.
7. Serve hot, and squeeze a lemon wedge over each bowl before enjoying this nutritious Spinach and White Bean Soup.

Mushroom and Barley Soup

Ingredients:

- 1 cup pearl barley, rinsed and drained
- 8 oz mushrooms, sliced
- 1 onion, finely chopped
- 3 cloves garlic, minced
- 4 cups vegetable broth
- 2 carrots, diced
- 2 celery stalks, chopped
- 1 teaspoon dried thyme
- Salt and pepper to taste
- Olive oil for sautéing
- Fresh parsley for garnish

Instructions:

1. In a pot, sauté the chopped onion in olive oil over medium heat until translucent.
2. Add minced garlic and cook for an additional minute until fragrant.
3. Stir in sliced mushrooms, diced carrots, and chopped celery.
4. Add pearl barley and vegetable broth to the pot.
5. Bring the soup to a boil, then reduce the heat to low, cover, and simmer for 25-30 minutes or until barley is tender.

6. Season with dried thyme, salt, and pepper to taste.

7. Ladle the soup into bowls and garnish with fresh parsley.

8. Enjoy this Mushroom and Barley Soup as a hearty and easy-to-make option.

Chickpea and Vegetable Stew

Ingredients:

- 1 can (15 oz) chickpeas, drained and rinsed
- 4 cups vegetable broth
- 1 onion, finely chopped
- 2 carrots, diced
- 2 zucchinis, sliced
- 1 can (14 oz) diced tomatoes
- 3 cloves garlic, minced
- 1 teaspoon dried Italian herbs
- Salt and pepper to taste
- Olive oil for sautéing
- Fresh basil for garnish

Instructions:

1. In a pot, sauté the chopped onion in olive oil over medium heat until translucent.

2. Add minced garlic and cook for an additional minute until fragrant.

3. Stir in diced carrots, sliced zucchinis, and cook for a few minutes until they begin to soften.

4. Add chickpeas, diced tomatoes (with their juices), and vegetable broth to the pot.

5. Bring the stew to a boil, then reduce the heat to low, cover, and simmer for 15-20 minutes.

6. Season with dried Italian herbs, salt, and pepper to taste.

7. Ladle the stew into bowls and garnish with fresh basil.

8. Serve this Chickpea and Vegetable Stew and enjoy!

Quinoa and Vegetable Soup

Ingredients:

- 1 cup quinoa, rinsed and drained
- 4 cups vegetable broth
- 1 onion, finely chopped
- 2 carrots, sliced
- 1 bell pepper, diced
- 1 can (14 oz) diced tomatoes
- 3 cloves garlic, minced

- 1 teaspoon ground cumin
- 1 teaspoon dried thyme
- Salt and pepper to taste
- Olive oil for sautéing
- Fresh parsley for garnish

Instructions:

1. In a pot, sauté the chopped onion in olive oil over medium heat until translucent.
2. Add minced garlic and cook for an additional minute until fragrant.
3. Stir in sliced carrots, diced bell pepper, and cook for a few minutes until slightly softened.
4. Add quinoa, diced tomatoes (with their juices), vegetable broth, ground cumin, and dried thyme to the pot.
5. Bring the soup to a boil, then reduce the heat to low, cover, and simmer for 15-20 minutes or until quinoa is cooked.
6. Season with salt and pepper to taste.
7. Ladle the soup into bowls and garnish with fresh parsley.
8. Serve and enjoy this Quinoa and Vegetable Soup.

Red Lentil and Tomato Soup

Ingredients:

- 1 cup red lentils, rinsed and drained
- 1 can (14 oz) diced tomatoes
- 1 onion, finely chopped
- 3 cloves garlic, minced
- 4 cups vegetable broth
- 1 teaspoon ground cumin
- 1/2 teaspoon smoked paprika
- Salt and pepper to taste
- Olive oil for sautéing
- Fresh cilantro for garnish

Instructions:

1. In a pot, sauté the chopped onion in olive oil over medium heat until translucent.
2. Add minced garlic and cook for an additional minute until fragrant.
3. Stir in red lentils, diced tomatoes (with their juices), vegetable broth, ground cumin, and smoked paprika.
4. Bring the soup to a boil, then reduce the heat to low, cover, and simmer for 15-20 minutes or until lentils are tender.
5. Season with salt and pepper to taste.

6. Ladle the soup into bowls and garnish with fresh cilantro.

7. Serve this Red Lentil and Tomato Soup and enjoy

Black Bean and Corn Chowder

Ingredients:

- 2 cans (15 oz each) black beans, drained and rinsed
- 1 cup frozen corn kernels
- 1 onion, finely chopped
- 2 cloves garlic, minced
- 4 cups vegetable broth
- 1 cup milk (or plant-based milk for a dairy-free option)
- 1 teaspoon ground cumin
- 1/2 teaspoon chili powder
- Salt and pepper to taste
- Olive oil for sautéing
- Fresh cilantro for garnish

Instructions:

1. In a pot, sauté the chopped onion in olive oil over medium heat until translucent.

2. Add minced garlic and cook for an additional minute until fragrant.

3. Stir in black beans, frozen corn, vegetable broth, ground cumin, and chili powder.

4. Bring the chowder to a simmer, then reduce the heat to low, cover, and let it cook for 15-20 minutes.

5. Pour in the milk and stir until well combined. Simmer for an additional 5 minutes.

6. Season with salt and pepper to taste.

7. Ladle the chowder into bowls and garnish with fresh cilantro.

8. Serve this Black Bean and Corn Chowder and enjoy.

Vegetable and Lentil Curry Soup

Ingredients:

- 1 cup dried green or brown lentils, rinsed and drained
- 1 can (14 oz) coconut milk
- 1 onion, finely chopped
- 2 carrots, diced
- 1 bell pepper, sliced
- 3 cloves garlic, minced

- 1 tablespoon curry powder
- 4 cups vegetable broth
- Salt and pepper to taste
- Olive oil for sautéing
- Fresh cilantro for garnish

Instructions:

1. In a pot, sauté the chopped onion in olive oil over medium heat until translucent.
2. Add minced garlic and cook for an additional minute until fragrant.
3. Stir in diced carrots, sliced bell pepper, and cook for a few minutes until slightly softened.
4. Add dried lentils, curry powder, coconut milk, and vegetable broth to the pot.
5. Bring the soup to a boil, then reduce the heat to low, cover, and simmer for 20-25 minutes or until lentils are tender.
6. Season with salt and pepper to taste.
7. Ladle the soup into bowls and garnish with fresh cilantro.
8. Serve and enjoy this Vegetable and Lentil Curry Soup.

CHAPTER 9: FISH AND POULTRY DISHES FOR FIBROID HEALTH

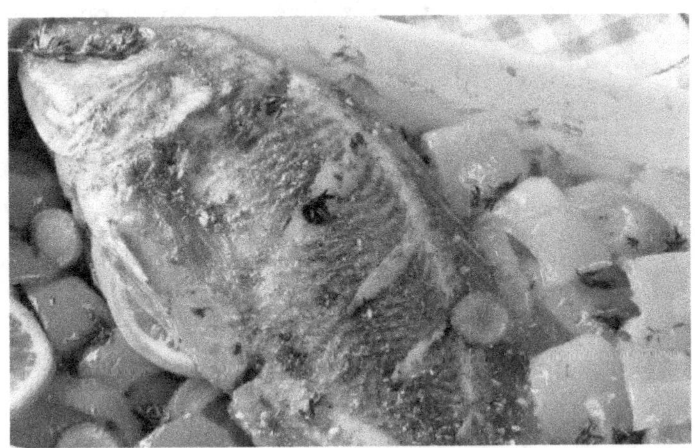

Baked Lemon Herb Tilapia

Ingredients:

- 4 tilapia filets
- 2 tablespoons olive oil
- 2 tablespoons fresh lemon juice
- 1 teaspoon dried oregano
- 1 teaspoon dried thyme
- 1 teaspoon garlic powder
- Salt and pepper to taste
- Lemon slices for garnish
- Fresh parsley for garnish

Instructions:

1. Preheat the oven to 400°F (200°C).

2. Place tilapia filets in a baking dish.

3. In a small bowl, mix olive oil, fresh lemon juice, dried oregano, dried thyme, and garlic powder.

4. Drizzle the mixture over the tilapia filets, ensuring they are well coated.

5. Season with salt and pepper to taste.

6. Bake in the preheated oven for 15-20 minutes or until the tilapia is opaque and flakes easily with a fork.

7. Garnish with lemon slices and fresh parsley before serving.

8. Serve and enjoy this Baked Lemon Herb Tilapia.

Lemon Garlic Baked Chicken Breast

Ingredients:

- 4 boneless, skinless chicken breasts
- 3 tablespoons olive oil
- 3 cloves garlic, minced
- 1 teaspoon dried thyme
- Zest of 1 lemon
- Juice of 1 lemon
- Salt and pepper to taste

- Fresh parsley for garnish

Instructions:

1. Preheat the oven to 400°F (200°C).

2. In a small bowl, mix olive oil, minced garlic, dried thyme, lemon zest, and lemon juice.

3. Place the chicken breasts in a baking dish and season them with salt and pepper.

4. Pour the lemon garlic mixture over the chicken breasts, ensuring they are well coated.

5. Bake in the preheated oven for 20-25 minutes or until the chicken is cooked through and no longer pink in the center.

6. Optionally, broil for an additional 2-3 minutes for a golden finish.

7. Garnish with fresh parsley before serving.

8. Serve this Lemon Garlic Baked Chicken Breast and enjoy!

Grilled Lemon Herb Chicken Skewers

Ingredients:

- 1.5 lbs boneless, skinless chicken breasts, cut into cubes
- 2 tablespoons olive oil
- Zest of 1 lemon

- Juice of 1 lemon
- 1 teaspoon dried rosemary
- 1 teaspoon dried thyme
- Salt and pepper to taste
- Wooden skewers, soaked in water for 30 minutes
- Fresh parsley for garnish

Instructions:

1. In a bowl, mix olive oil, lemon zest, lemon juice, dried rosemary, dried thyme, salt, and pepper.
2. Thread the chicken cubes onto the soaked skewers.
3. Brush the chicken skewers with the lemon herb mixture, ensuring they are well coated.
4. Preheat the grill to medium-high heat.
5. Grill the chicken skewers for 8-10 minutes, turning occasionally, until the chicken is cooked through and has a nice char.
6. Remove from the grill and garnish with fresh parsley.
7. Serve these Grilled Lemon Herb Chicken Skewers and enjoy.

Honey Mustard Salmon

Ingredients:

- 4 salmon filets
- 3 tablespoons Dijon mustard
- 2 tablespoons honey
- 1 tablespoon olive oil
- 1 teaspoon garlic powder
- Salt and pepper to taste
- Fresh dill for garnish

Instructions:

1. Preheat the oven to 400°F (200°C).
2. Place salmon filets on a baking sheet lined with parchment paper.
3. In a small bowl, mix Dijon mustard, honey, olive oil, garlic powder, salt, and pepper.
4. Brush the honey mustard mixture over the salmon filets, ensuring they are well coated.
5. Bake in the preheated oven for 12-15 minutes or until the salmon is flaky and cooked to your liking.
6. Garnish with fresh dill before serving.
7. Serve and enjoy this Honey Mustard Salmon.

Herb-Roasted Turkey Breast

Ingredients:

- 1 boneless, skinless turkey breast (about 2 lbs)
- 2 tablespoons olive oil
- 1 teaspoon dried sage
- 1 teaspoon dried thyme
- 1 teaspoon dried rosemary
- Salt and pepper to taste
- 2 cloves garlic, minced
- Fresh parsley for garnish

Instructions:

1. Preheat the oven to 375°F (190°C).
2. Place the turkey breast in a roasting pan or on a baking sheet.
3. In a small bowl, mix olive oil, dried sage, dried thyme, dried rosemary, salt, pepper, and minced garlic.
4. Rub the herb mixture over the turkey breast, ensuring it's evenly coated.
5. Roast in the preheated oven for approximately 50-60 minutes or until the internal temperature reaches 165°F (74°C).
6. Allow the turkey breast to rest for 10 minutes before slicing.

7. Garnish with fresh parsley before serving.

8. Serve this Herb-Roasted Turkey Breast and enjoy.

Lemon Garlic Shrimp Skillet

Ingredients:

- 1 lb large shrimp, peeled and deveined
- 2 tablespoons olive oil
- 3 cloves garlic, minced
- Zest of 1 lemon
- Juice of 1 lemon
- 1 teaspoon dried oregano
- Salt and pepper to taste
- Fresh parsley for garnish

Instructions:

1. In a large skillet, heat olive oil over medium heat.

2. Add minced garlic and sauté for about 1 minute until fragrant.

3. Add the shrimp to the skillet, cooking for 2-3 minutes on each side until they turn pink and opaque.

4. Stir in lemon zest, lemon juice, dried oregano, salt, and pepper.

5. Cook for an additional 2 minutes, ensuring the shrimp are well-coated in the lemon garlic mixture.

6. Garnish with fresh parsley before serving.

7. Serve this Lemon Garlic Shrimp Skillet and enjoy!

Baked Dijon Mustard Cod

Ingredients:

- 4 cod filets
- 3 tablespoons Dijon mustard
- 2 tablespoons olive oil
- 1 tablespoon lemon juice
- 1 teaspoon dried thyme
- Salt and pepper to taste
- Fresh chives for garnish

Instructions:

1. Preheat the oven to 400°F (200°C).

2. Place cod filets on a baking sheet lined with parchment paper.

3. In a small bowl, whisk together Dijon mustard, olive oil, lemon juice, dried thyme, salt, and pepper.

4. Brush the Dijon mustard mixture over the cod filets, ensuring they are well coated.

5. Bake in the preheated oven for 12-15 minutes or until the cod is flaky and cooked through.

6. Garnish with fresh chives before serving.

7. Serve and enjoy this Baked Dijon Mustard.

One-Pan Lemon Garlic Chicken Thighs with Vegetables

Ingredients:

- 4 bone-in, skin-on chicken thighs
- 1 lb baby potatoes, halved
- 1 cup baby carrots
- 1 tablespoon olive oil
- 3 cloves garlic, minced
- Zest of 1 lemon
- Juice of 1 lemon
- 1 teaspoon dried rosemary
- Salt and pepper to taste
- Fresh parsley for garnish

Instructions:

1. Preheat the oven to 425°F (220°C).

2. In a large bowl, toss halved baby potatoes and baby carrots with olive oil, minced garlic, lemon zest, dried rosemary, salt, and pepper.

3. Place the chicken thighs on a baking sheet and arrange the seasoned vegetables around them.

4. Drizzle lemon juice over the chicken and vegetables.

5. Roast in the preheated oven for 30-35 minutes or until the chicken is golden brown and the vegetables are tender.

6. Garnish with fresh parsley before serving.

7. Serve and enjoy this One-Pan Lemon Garlic Chicken Thighs with Vegetables.

Baked Lemon Butter Salmon

Ingredients:

- 4 salmon filets
- 3 tablespoons melted butter
- 2 tablespoons fresh lemon juice
- 1 teaspoon garlic powder
- Salt and pepper to taste
- Lemon slices for garnish
- Fresh dill for garnish

Instructions:

1. Preheat the oven to 400°F (200°C).
2. Place salmon filets on a baking sheet lined with parchment paper.
3. In a small bowl, mix melted butter, fresh lemon juice, garlic powder, salt, and pepper.
4. Brush the lemon butter mixture over the salmon filets, ensuring they are well coated.
5. Place a lemon slice on top of each filet for added flavor.
6. Bake in the preheated oven for 12-15 minutes or until the salmon is flaky and cooked to your liking.
7. Garnish with fresh dill before serving.
8. Serve this Baked Lemon Butter Salmon and enjoy.

Teriyaki Chicken Stir-Fry

Ingredients:

- 1 lb boneless, skinless chicken breasts, thinly sliced
- 2 cups broccoli florets
- 1 red bell pepper, thinly sliced
- 1 cup snap peas, ends trimmed

- 3 tablespoons soy sauce
- 2 tablespoons honey
- 1 tablespoon sesame oil
- 1 teaspoon minced ginger
- 2 cloves garlic, minced
- 2 tablespoons vegetable oil
- Sesame seeds for garnish (optional)
- Cooked brown rice for serving

Instructions:

1. In a small bowl, whisk together soy sauce, honey, sesame oil, minced ginger, and minced garlic to create the teriyaki sauce.
2. Heat vegetable oil in a large skillet or wok over medium-high heat.
3. Add sliced chicken to the skillet and cook until browned and cooked through.
4. Add broccoli, red bell pepper, and snap peas to the skillet, stirring continuously for 3-5 minutes until the vegetables are tender-crisp.
5. Pour the teriyaki sauce over the chicken and vegetables, tossing to coat evenly.
6. Cook for an additional 2-3 minutes until everything is well combined and heated through.

7. Serve the Teriyaki Chicken Stir-Fry over cooked brown rice.

8. Optionally, garnish with sesame seeds for added texture.

9. Serve and enjoy this Teriyaki Chicken Stir-Fry.

Baked Pesto Chicken

Ingredients:

- 4 boneless, skinless chicken breasts
- 1/2 cup pesto sauce (store-bought or homemade)
- 1 cup cherry tomatoes, halved
- 1 cup mozzarella cheese, shredded
- Salt and pepper to taste
- Fresh basil leaves for garnish

Instructions:

1. Preheat the oven to 400°F (200°C).

2. Place chicken breasts in a baking dish and season with salt and pepper.

3. Spread a generous layer of pesto sauce over each chicken breast.

4. Arrange halved cherry tomatoes on top of the pesto-covered chicken.

5. Sprinkle shredded mozzarella cheese over the tomatoes.

6. Bake in the preheated oven for 20-25 minutes or until the chicken is cooked through, and the cheese is melted and bubbly.

7. Garnish with fresh basil leaves before serving.

8. Serve this Baked Pesto Chicken and enjoy!

Lemon Herb Grilled Turkey Burgers

Ingredients:

- 1 lb ground turkey
- 1 tablespoon olive oil
- Zest of 1 lemon
- 1 teaspoon dried oregano
- 1 teaspoon dried thyme
- Salt and pepper to taste
- Whole wheat burger buns
- Lettuce, tomato, and red onion slices for topping

Instructions:

1. Preheat the grill to medium-high heat.

2. In a bowl, combine ground turkey, olive oil, lemon zest, dried oregano, dried thyme, salt, and pepper. Mix until well combined.

3. Divide the turkey mixture into equal portions and shape into burger patties.

4. Grill the turkey burgers for approximately 5-6 minutes per side or until fully cooked.

5. Toast the whole wheat burger buns on the grill for a minute or two.

6. Assemble the burgers with lettuce, tomato, and red onion slices.

7. Serve these Lemon Herb Grilled Turkey Burgers and enjoy.

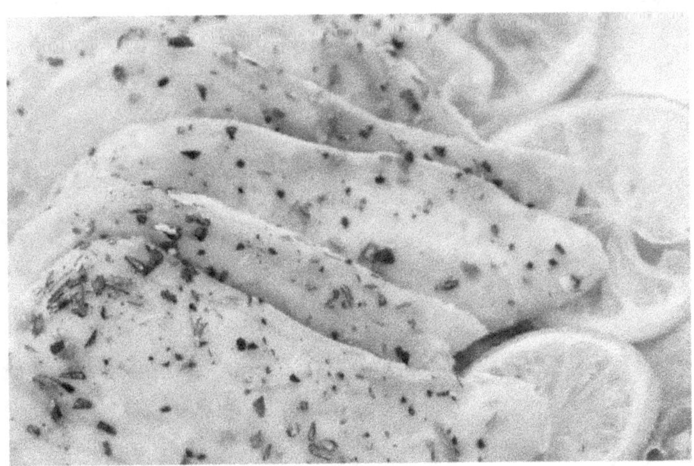

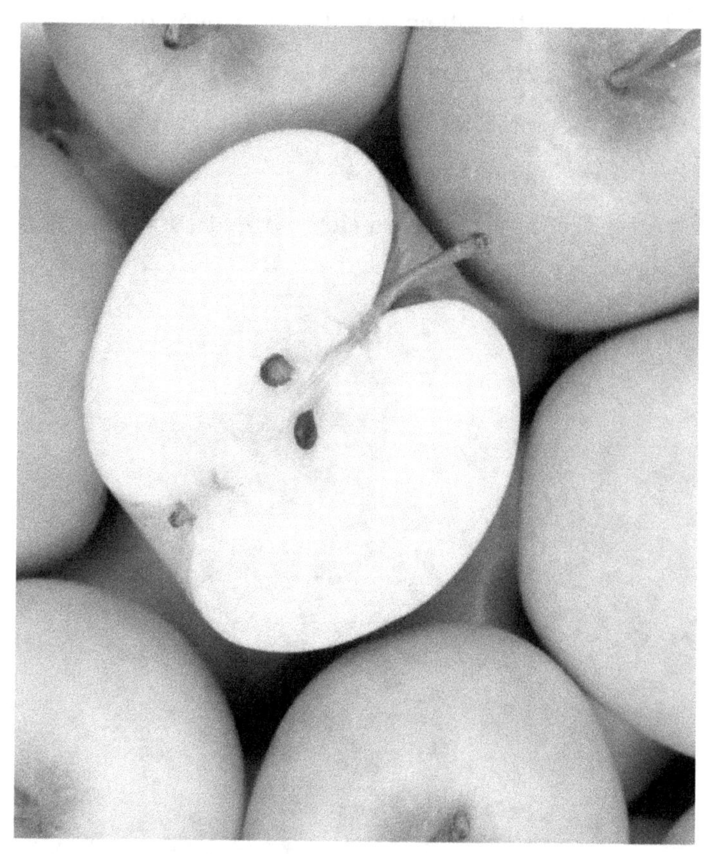

CHAPTER 10: HERBS AND SPICES

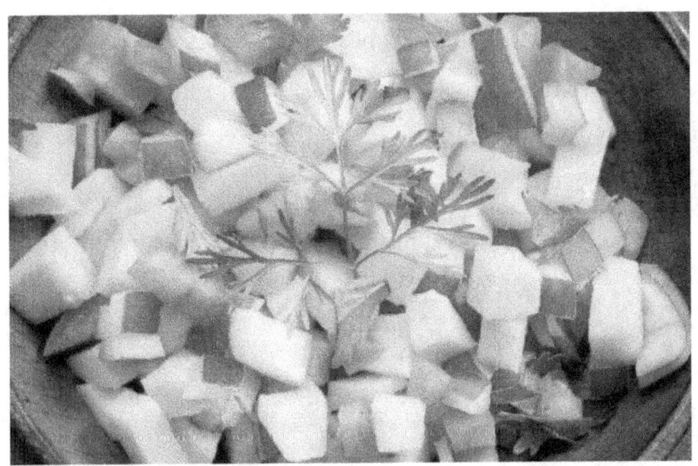

Mango Basil Salsa

Ingredients:

- 2 ripe mangoes, diced
- 1/2 red onion, finely chopped
- 1/4 cup fresh basil, thinly sliced
- Juice of 1 lime
- 1 small jalapeño, seeded and finely chopped
- Salt and pepper to taste

Instructions:

1. In a bowl, combine diced mangoes, finely chopped red onion, sliced fresh basil, and chopped jalapeño.

2. Squeeze the juice of one lime over the mixture.

3. Toss gently to combine all the ingredients.

4. Season with salt and pepper to taste.

5. Allow the salsa to sit for 15-20 minutes to let the flavors meld.

6. Serve this Mango Basil Salsa as a vibrant and easy-to-make topping for grilled chicken, fish, or as a refreshing dip for whole-grain tortilla chips.

Garlic Herb Quinoa

Ingredients:

- 1 cup quinoa, rinsed
- 2 cups vegetable broth
- 2 cloves garlic, minced
- 1 tablespoon olive oil
- 1 teaspoon dried basil
- 1 teaspoon dried thyme
- Salt and pepper to taste
- Fresh parsley for garnish

Instructions:

1. In a medium saucepan, heat olive oil over medium heat.

2. Add minced garlic and sauté for 1 minute until fragrant.

3. Add rinsed quinoa to the saucepan, stirring to coat the quinoa in the garlic-infused oil.

4. Pour in the vegetable broth, add dried basil and dried thyme, and season with salt and pepper.

5. Bring the mixture to a boil, then reduce the heat to low, cover, and simmer for 15-20 minutes or until the quinoa is cooked and the liquid is absorbed.

6. Fluff the quinoa with a fork and let it sit covered for an additional 5 minutes.

7. Garnish with fresh parsley before serving.

8. Serve and enjoy this Garlic Herb Quinoa.

Turmeric Ginger Infused Detox Water

Ingredients:

- 1 teaspoon ground turmeric
- 1 teaspoon fresh ginger, grated
- 1 lemon, thinly sliced
- 1 cucumber, thinly sliced
- 1-2 sprigs of fresh mint
- 4 cups water
- Ice cubes (optional)

Instructions:

1. In a pitcher, combine ground turmeric and grated fresh ginger.
2. Add thinly sliced lemon and cucumber to the pitcher.
3. Place mint sprigs on top of the other ingredients.
4. Pour 4 cups of water into the pitcher.
5. Stir gently to mix the ingredients.
6. Refrigerate for at least 2 hours to allow the flavors to infuse.
7. Serve over ice cubes if desired.
8. Serve and enjoy this Turmeric Ginger Infused Detox Water.

Lemon Rosemary Roasted Chickpeas

Ingredients:

- 1 can (15 oz) chickpeas, drained and rinsed
- 2 tablespoons olive oil
- Zest of 1 lemon
- 1 teaspoon dried rosemary
- 1/2 teaspoon garlic powder
- Salt and pepper to taste

Instructions:

1. Preheat the oven to 400°F (200°C).

2. Pat the chickpeas dry with a paper towel.

3. In a bowl, toss chickpeas with olive oil, lemon zest, dried rosemary, garlic powder, salt, and pepper.

4. Spread the seasoned chickpeas in a single layer on a baking sheet.

5. Roast in the preheated oven for 20-25 minutes or until the chickpeas are golden and crispy.

6. Allow them to cool for a few minutes before serving.

7. Enjoy these Lemon Rosemary Roasted Chickpeas!

Chili Lime Avocado Toast

Ingredients:

- 2 slices whole-grain bread
- 1 ripe avocado
- Juice of 1 lime
- 1/2 teaspoon chili powder
- Salt and pepper to taste
- Fresh cilantro for garnish (optional)

Instructions:

1. Toast the whole-grain bread slices.

2. In a bowl, mash the ripe avocado with lime juice, chili powder, salt, and pepper.

3. Spread the avocado mixture evenly over the toasted bread slices.

4. Garnish with fresh cilantro if desired.

5. Serve this Chili Lime Avocado Toast as a quick, zesty, and herb-infused breakfast or snack.

Minty Cucumber Yogurt Dip

Ingredients:

- 1 cup Greek yogurt
- 1 cucumber, finely diced
- 2 tablespoons fresh mint, chopped
- 1 clove garlic, minced
- 1 tablespoon lemon juice
- Salt and pepper to taste

Instructions:

1. In a bowl, combine Greek yogurt, finely diced cucumber, chopped fresh mint, minced garlic, lemon juice, salt, and pepper.

2. Mix the ingredients until well combined.

3. Refrigerate for at least 30 minutes to let the flavors meld.

4. Stir again before serving.

5. Use this Minty Cucumber Yogurt Dip as a refreshing and easy-to-make accompaniment for veggies, pita chips, or as a light dressing for salads.

Basil Lime Quinoa Salad

Ingredients:

- 1 cup quinoa, cooked and cooled
- 1 cup cherry tomatoes, halved
- 1/2 cup fresh basil leaves, chopped
- Zest and juice of 1 lime
- 2 tablespoons olive oil
- Salt and pepper to taste

Instructions:

1. In a large bowl, combine cooked and cooled quinoa, cherry tomatoes, and chopped fresh basil.
2. In a small bowl, whisk together lime zest, lime juice, olive oil, salt, and pepper.
3. Pour the dressing over the quinoa mixture and toss until well combined.
4. Refrigerate for at least 30 minutes to let the flavors meld.

5. Serve this Basil Lime Quinoa Salad as a light,
    herb-infused side dish or a standalone meal.

Lemon Dill Salmon Packets

Ingredients:

- 2 salmon filets
- Zest and juice of 1 lemon
- 2 tablespoons fresh dill, chopped
- 1 tablespoon olive oil
- Salt and pepper to taste
- Sliced lemon for garnish

Instructions:

1. Preheat the oven to 375°F (190°C).
2. Place each salmon filet on a piece of aluminum foil.
3. In a small bowl, mix together lemon zest, lemon juice, chopped fresh dill, olive oil, salt, and pepper.
4. Spoon the lemon-dill mixture over each salmon filet.
5. Fold the aluminum foil around the salmon to create a packet, ensuring it's well-sealed.
6. Bake in the preheated oven for 15-20 minutes or until the salmon is cooked through.

7. Carefully open the foil packets, garnish with sliced lemon, and serve.

8. Enjoy these Lemon Dill Salmon Packets as a quick, herb-infused, and healthy fish dish.

Herb-Infused Quinoa Stuffed Bell Peppers

Ingredients:

- 4 bell peppers, halved and seeds removed
- 1 cup quinoa, cooked
- 1 can (15 oz) black beans, drained and rinsed
- 1 cup corn kernels (fresh, frozen, or canned)
- 1 teaspoon cumin
- 1 teaspoon dried oregano
- Salt and pepper to taste
- Fresh cilantro for garnish

Instructions:

1. Preheat the oven to 375°F (190°C).

2. In a large bowl, combine cooked quinoa, black beans, corn, cumin, dried oregano, salt, and pepper.

3. Stuff each bell pepper half with the quinoa mixture.

4. Place the stuffed peppers in a baking dish.

5. Bake in the preheated oven for 25-30 minutes or until the peppers are tender.

6. Garnish with fresh cilantro before serving.

7. Enjoy these Herb-Infused Quinoa Stuffed Bell Peppers as a flavorful, herb-infused, and easy-to-make dish.

Garlic Herb Zucchini Noodles

Ingredients:

- 4 medium-sized zucchinis
- 2 tablespoons olive oil
- 3 cloves garlic, minced
- 1 teaspoon dried Italian herbs (basil, oregano, thyme)
- Salt and pepper to taste
- Grated Parmesan cheese for garnish (optional)

Instructions:

1. Using a spiralizer or a vegetable peeler, create zucchini noodles from the zucchinis.

2. Heat olive oil in a large skillet over medium heat.

3. Add minced garlic to the skillet and sauté for 1-2 minutes until fragrant.

4. Add zucchini noodles to the skillet and toss to coat them in the garlic-infused oil.

5. Sprinkle dried Italian herbs over the noodles and continue to sauté for 3-4 minutes or until the noodles are tender but still crisp.

6. Season with salt and pepper to taste.

7. Garnish with grated Parmesan cheese if desired.

8. Serve these Garlic Herb Zucchini Noodles as a quick, low-carb, and herb-infused alternative to traditional pasta.

Cilantro Lime Cauliflower Rice

Ingredients:

- 1 head cauliflower, grated or processed into rice-like texture
- 2 tablespoons olive oil
- 1/4 cup fresh cilantro, chopped
- Zest and juice of 1 lime
- Salt and pepper to taste

Instructions:

1. In a large skillet, heat olive oil over medium heat.

2. Add the cauliflower rice to the skillet and sauté for 5-7 minutes until it starts to soften.

3. Stir in chopped cilantro and continue to sauté for an additional 2-3 minutes.

4. Add lime zest and lime juice to the cauliflower rice, mixing well.

5. Season with salt and pepper to taste.

6. Cook for another 2-3 minutes until the cauliflower rice is tender but not mushy.

7. Serve this Cilantro Lime Cauliflower Rice as a flavorful, low-carb, and herb-infused side dish.

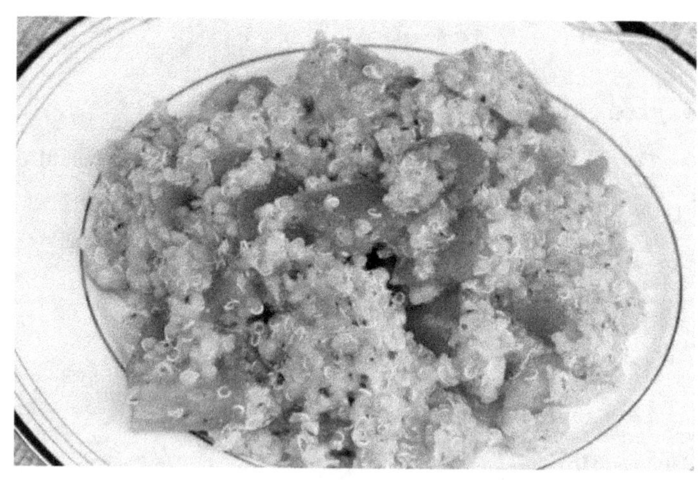

CHAPTER 11: HERBAL TEAS FOR UTERINE HEALTH

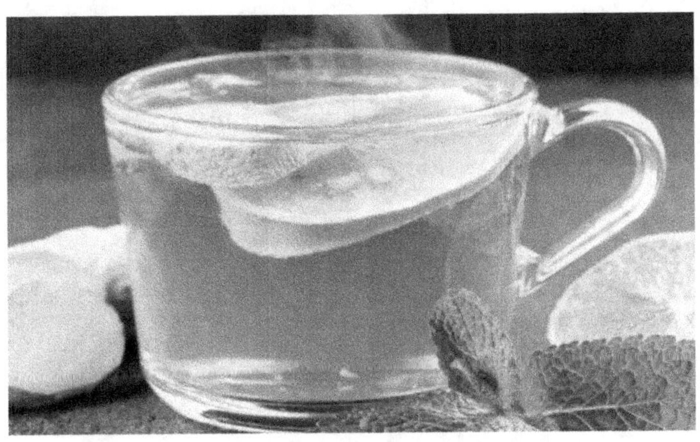

Ginger Mint Herbal Tea

Ingredients:

- 1-inch piece of fresh ginger, thinly sliced
- 1 bunch fresh mint leaves
- 4 cups water
- Honey (optional, for sweetness)

Instructions:

1. In a pot, bring 4 cups of water to a gentle boil.
2. Add thinly sliced ginger to the boiling water.
3. Tear the fresh mint leaves and add them to the pot.

4. Reduce the heat and let the tea simmer for 5-7 minutes.

5. Remove the pot from heat and strain the tea to remove ginger and mint leaves.

6. Pour the tea into your favorite mug.

7. Add honey if desired for sweetness.

8. Enjoy this Ginger Mint Herbal Tea as a soothing and herb-infused beverage.

Chamomile Lavender Sleepy Tea

Ingredients:

- 2 chamomile tea bags
- 1 teaspoon dried lavender flowers (culinary-grade)
- 4 cups hot water
- Lemon or honey (optional, for flavor)

Instructions:

1. Place chamomile tea bags and dried lavender flowers in a teapot or heatproof pitcher.

2. Pour hot water over the tea bags and lavender.

3. Let it steep for 5-7 minutes, allowing the calming aromas to infuse into the water.

4. Remove the tea bags and lavender from the pot.

5. Pour the tea into your favorite cup.

6. Add a splash of lemon or honey if desired for extra flavor.

7. Sip and unwind with this Chamomile Lavender Sleepy Tea as a calming and easy-to-make herbal infusion for relaxation.

Rosemary Lemon Infusion

Ingredients:

- 2 sprigs fresh rosemary
- 1 lemon, thinly sliced
- 4 cups hot water
- Optional: Honey for sweetness

Instructions:

1. Place fresh rosemary sprigs and lemon slices in a teapot or heatproof pitcher.
2. Pour hot water over the rosemary and lemon.
3. Let it steep for 5-7 minutes to infuse the flavors.
4. Remove the rosemary sprigs and lemon slices.
5. Pour the aromatic infusion into your cup.
6. Add honey if desired for a touch of sweetness.
7. Enjoy this Rosemary Lemon Infusion as a refreshing and easy-to-make herbal tea.

Cinnamon Apple Spice Tea

Ingredients:

- 2 cinnamon sticks
- 1 apple, thinly sliced
- 4 cups hot water
- Optional: a dash of ground cinnamon
- Optional: Honey for sweetness

Instructions:

1. Place cinnamon sticks and thinly sliced apple in a teapot or heatproof pitcher.
2. Pour hot water over the cinnamon sticks and apple slices.
3. Allow the tea to steep for 5-7 minutes, letting the cinnamon and apple flavors meld.
4. Remove the cinnamon sticks and apple slices.
5. Pour the fragrant tea into your cup.
6. Add a dash of ground cinnamon for extra warmth if desired.
7. Sweeten with honey if you prefer a sweeter taste.
8. Savor this Cinnamon Apple Spice Tea as a delightful and easy-to-make herbal beverage.

Turmeric Ginger Citrus Tea

Ingredients:

- 1 teaspoon ground turmeric
- 1 teaspoon fresh ginger, grated
- 1 orange, sliced
- 4 cups hot water
- Optional: a squeeze of lemon juice
- Optional: Honey for sweetness

Instructions:

1. Combine ground turmeric and freshly grated ginger in a teapot or heatproof pitcher.
2. Add orange slices to the mixture.
3. Pour hot water over the turmeric, ginger, and orange.
4. Let it steep for 5-7 minutes, allowing the vibrant flavors to infuse.
5. Remove the orange slices.
6. Squeeze a bit of lemon juice for a citrusy kick if desired.
7. Sweeten with honey to taste.
8. Enjoy this Turmeric Ginger Citrus Tea as a zesty and easy-to-make herbal concoction.

Peppermint Rose Hibiscus Tea

Ingredients:

- 2 peppermint tea bags
- 1 tablespoon dried rose petals
- 1 tablespoon dried hibiscus petals
- 4 cups hot water
- Optional: Fresh mint leaves for garnish

Instructions:

1. Place peppermint tea bags, dried rose petals, and dried hibiscus petals in a teapot or heatproof pitcher.
2. Pour hot water over the tea bags and petals.
3. Let it steep for 5-7 minutes, allowing the vibrant colors and refreshing flavors to mingle.
4. Remove the tea bags and petals.
5. Pour the aromatic infusion into your cup.
6. Garnish with fresh mint leaves for an extra burst of freshness if desired.
7. Sip and relish this Peppermint Rose Hibiscus Tea as a delightful and easy-to-make herbal blend.

Lemon Basil Green Tea

Ingredients:

- 2 green tea bags
- 1 lemon, sliced
- 1/4 cup fresh basil leaves
- 4 cups hot water
- Optional: Honey for sweetness

Instructions:

1. Place green tea bags, lemon slices, and fresh basil leaves in a teapot or heatproof pitcher.
2. Pour hot water over the tea bags, lemon, and basil.
3. Let it steep for 3-5 minutes, allowing the green tea to infuse with citrusy and herbal notes.
4. Remove the tea bags, lemon slices, and basil leaves.
5. Pour the fragrant tea into your cup.
6. Sweeten with honey if desired.
7. Enjoy this Lemon Basil Green Tea as a refreshing and easy-to-make herbal beverage.

Mango Ginger Mint Tea

Ingredients:

- 1 black tea bag
- 1/2 cup ripe mango, diced
- 1 teaspoon fresh ginger, grated
- 4-5 fresh mint leaves
- 4 cups hot water
- Optional: Honey for sweetness

Instructions:

1. Place the black tea bag, diced mango, grated ginger, and fresh mint leaves in a teapot or heatproof pitcher.
2. Pour hot water over the tea bag, mango, ginger, and mint.
3. Let it steep for 4-6 minutes, allowing the flavors to meld.
4. Remove the tea bag and strain the tea to remove mango, ginger, and mint leaves.
5. Pour the infused tea into your cup.
6. Sweeten with honey if desired.
7. Enjoy this Mango Ginger Mint Tea as a tropical and easy-to-make herbal blend.

Lavender Blueberry Bliss Tea

Ingredients:

- 2 herbal blueberry tea bags
- 1 tablespoon dried lavender buds
- 1/2 cup fresh blueberries
- 4 cups hot water
- Optional: Lemon wedge for garnish

Instructions:

1. Place herbal blueberry tea bags, dried lavender buds, and fresh blueberries in a teapot or heatproof pitcher.
2. Pour hot water over the tea bags, lavender, and blueberries.
3. Let it steep for 5-7 minutes, allowing the fragrant blend to infuse.
4. Remove the tea bags and strain to remove lavender buds and blueberries.
5. Pour the vibrant tea into your cup.
6. Garnish with a lemon wedge if desired.
7. Sip and savor this Lavender Blueberry Bliss Tea as a delightful and easy-to-make herbal infusion.

Peach Rosemary Iced Tea

Ingredients:

- 2 black tea bags
- 1 peach, sliced
- 2 sprigs fresh rosemary
- 4 cups hot water
- Ice cubes
- Optional: Honey for sweetness

Instructions:

1. Place black tea bags, sliced peach, and fresh rosemary sprigs in a heatproof pitcher.
2. Pour hot water over the tea bags, peach, and rosemary.
3. Let it steep for 4-6 minutes, allowing the flavors to meld.
4. Remove the tea bags and rosemary sprigs.
5. Allow the tea to cool, then refrigerate until cold.
6. Fill glasses with ice cubes and pour the chilled tea over.
7. Sweeten with honey if desired.
8. Enjoy this Peach Rosemary Iced Tea as a refreshing and easy-to-make herbal iced tea.

CHAPTER 12: SMOOTHIES

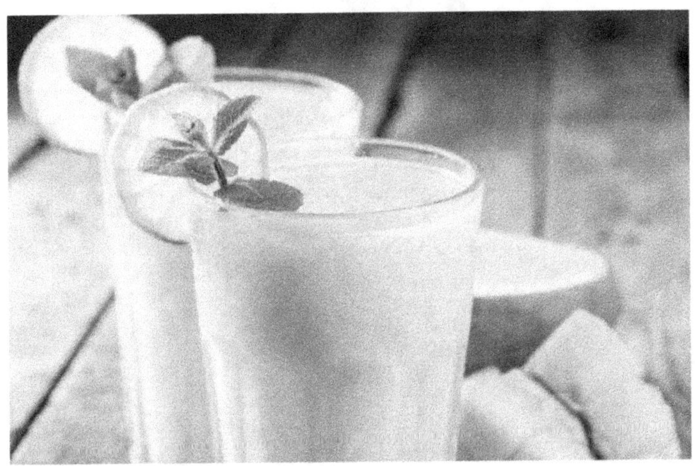

Minty Mango Avocado Smoothie

Ingredients:

- 1 cup ripe mango chunks
- 1/2 avocado
- Handful of fresh mint leaves
- 1 tablespoon hemp seeds
- 1 cup coconut water
- 1/2 lime, juiced
- Ice cubes

Instructions:

1. Combine ripe mango chunks, avocado, fresh mint leaves, hemp seeds, coconut water, and lime juice in a blender.

2. Blend until smooth and velvety.

3. Add ice cubes and blend again for a cool and refreshing texture.

4. Pour into a glass and enjoy this Minty Mango Avocado Smoothie.

Berry Bliss Smoothie

Ingredients:

- 1 cup mixed berries (strawberries, blueberries, raspberries)
- 1/2 banana
- 1/2 cup Greek yogurt
- 1 tablespoon chia seeds
- 1 cup spinach leaves
- 1/2 cup almond milk
- Ice cubes

Instructions:

1. Combine mixed berries, banana, Greek yogurt, chia seeds, spinach leaves, and almond milk in a blender.

2. Blend until smooth and creamy.

3. Add ice cubes and blend again until the desired consistency is reached.

4. Pour into a glass and enjoy this nutrient-packed Berry Bliss Smoothie.

Tropical Turmeric Pineapple Smoothie

Ingredients:

- 1 cup pineapple chunks
- 1/2 banana
- 1/2 teaspoon ground turmeric
- 1/2 teaspoon grated ginger
- 1 cup coconut water
- 1 tablespoon flaxseeds
- Ice cubes

Instructions:

1. Place pineapple chunks, banana, ground turmeric, grated ginger, coconut water, and flaxseeds in a blender.

2. Blend until smooth and creamy.

3. Add ice cubes and blend again for a refreshing chill.

4. Pour into a glass and enjoy this Tropical Turmeric Pineapple Smoothie.

Cucumber Kale Citrus Smoothie

Ingredients:

- 1/2 cucumber, peeled and sliced
- 1 cup kale leaves, stems removed
- 1 orange, peeled and segmented
- 1/2 banana
- 1 tablespoon chia seeds
- 1 cup coconut water
- Ice cubes

Instructions:

1. Combine cucumber slices, kale leaves, orange segments, banana, chia seeds, and coconut water in a blender.
2. Blend until smooth and vibrant.
3. Add ice cubes and blend again for a refreshing chill.
4. Pour into a glass and enjoy this Cucumber Kale Citrus Smoothie.

Pomegranate Green Tea Smoothie

Ingredients:

- 1/2 cup pomegranate seeds
- 1 green tea bag, brewed and cooled
- 1/2 cup pineapple chunks
- Handful of spinach leaves
- 1 tablespoon honey
- 1/2 lemon, juiced
- Ice cubes

Instructions:

1. Brew green tea and let it cool to room temperature.
2. In a blender, combine pomegranate seeds, cooled green tea, pineapple chunks, spinach leaves, honey, and lemon juice.
3. Blend until smooth and vibrant.
4. Add ice cubes and blend again for a cool and invigorating texture.
5. Pour into a glass and enjoy this Pomegranate Green Tea Smoothie.

Cherry Almond Protein Smoothie

Ingredients:

- 1 cup frozen cherries
- 1/2 cup plain Greek yogurt
- 1/4 cup almonds
- 1 tablespoon almond butter
- 1 scoop vanilla protein powder
- 1 cup almond milk
- Ice cubes

Instructions:

1. Combine frozen cherries, Greek yogurt, almonds, almond butter, vanilla protein powder, and almond milk in a blender.
2. Blend until smooth and creamy.
3. Add ice cubes and blend again for a refreshing chill.
4. Pour into a glass and enjoy this Cherry Almond Protein Smoothie.

Blueberry Basil Bliss Smoothie

Ingredients:

- 1 cup blueberries
- Handful of fresh basil leaves

- 1/2 cup cucumber, sliced
- 1/2 cup plain yogurt
- 1 tablespoon chia seeds
- 1 tablespoon honey
- 1 cup watermelon, cubed
- Ice cubes

Instructions:

1. In a blender, combine blueberries, fresh basil leaves, cucumber slices, plain yogurt, chia seeds, honey, and watermelon cubes.
2. Blend until smooth and aromatic.
3. Add ice cubes and blend again for a cool and refreshing texture.
4. Pour into a glass and enjoy this Blueberry Basil Bliss Smoothie.

Mango Matcha Madness Smoothie

Ingredients:

- 1 cup mango chunks
- 1 teaspoon matcha powder
- 1/2 cup cucumber, peeled and sliced
- 1 tablespoon flaxseeds
- 1/2 cup coconut milk
- 1 tablespoon agave nectar

- Ice cubes

Instructions:

1. Combine mango chunks, matcha powder, cucumber slices, flaxseeds, coconut milk, and agave nectar in a blender.
2. Blend until smooth and vibrant.
3. Add ice cubes and blend again for a refreshing chill.
4. Pour into a glass and enjoy this Mango Matcha Madness Smoothie.

Berry Beet Boost Smoothie

Ingredients:

- 1/2 cup mixed berries (strawberries, blueberries, raspberries)
- 1/2 small cooked beet, peeled and diced
- 1/2 cup Greek yogurt
- 1 tablespoon hemp seeds
- 1 tablespoon honey
- 1 cup almond milk
- Ice cubes

Instructions:

1. In a blender, combine mixed berries, cooked beet, Greek yogurt, hemp seeds, honey, and almond milk.
2. Blend until smooth and vibrant.
3. Add ice cubes and blend again for a refreshing chill.
4. Pour into a glass and enjoy this Berry Beet Boost Smoothie.

Turmeric Tropical Fusion Smoothie

Ingredients:

- 1 cup pineapple chunks
- 1/2 banana
- 1/2 teaspoon ground turmeric
- 1/2 teaspoon ginger, grated
- 1 tablespoon chia seeds
- 1 cup coconut water
- Ice cubes

Instructions:

1. Combine pineapple chunks, banana, ground turmeric, grated ginger, chia seeds, and coconut water in a blender.
2. Blend until smooth and vibrant.

3. Add ice cubes and blend again for a cool and exotic texture.

4. Pour into a glass and enjoy this Turmeric Tropical Fusion Smoothie.

Orange Carrot Citrus Splash Smoothie

Ingredients:

- 1 large orange, peeled and segmented
- 1 medium carrot, peeled and chopped
- 1/2 cup mango chunks
- 1 tablespoon flaxseeds
- 1/2 cup Greek yogurt
- 1 tablespoon honey
- 1 cup coconut water
- Ice cubes

Instructions:

1. In a blender, combine orange segments, chopped carrot, mango chunks, flaxseeds, Greek yogurt, honey, and coconut water.

2. Blend until smooth and citrusy.

3. Add ice cubes and blend again for a refreshing chill.

4. Pour into a glass and enjoy this Orange Carrot Citrus Splash Smoothie.

Pomegranate Mint Marvel Smoothie

Ingredients:

- 1 cup pomegranate seeds
- Handful of fresh mint leaves
- 1/2 cup cucumber, sliced
- 1/2 cup plain yogurt
- 1 tablespoon chia seeds
- 1 tablespoon maple syrup
- 1 cup coconut water
- Ice cubes

Instructions:

1. Combine pomegranate seeds, fresh mint leaves, cucumber slices, plain yogurt, chia seeds, maple syrup, and coconut water in a blender.
2. Blend until smooth and invigorating.
3. Add ice cubes and blend again for a crisp and delightful texture.
4. Pour into a glass and enjoy this Pomegranate Mint Marvel Smoothie.

Cherry Almond Delight Smoothie

Ingredients:

- 1 cup cherries, pitted

- 1/4 cup almonds, soaked and peeled
- 1/2 banana
- 1 tablespoon almond butter
- 1/2 cup Greek yogurt
- 1 tablespoon honey
- 1 cup almond milk
- Ice cubes

Instructions:

1. In a blender, combine pitted cherries, soaked almonds, banana, almond butter, Greek yogurt, honey, and almond milk.
2. Blend until smooth and luscious.
3. Add ice cubes and blend again for a cool and nutty texture.
4. Pour into a glass and enjoy this Cherry Almond Delight Smoothie.

Avocado Green Goddess Smoothie

Ingredients:

- 1/2 ripe avocado
- Handful of spinach leaves
- 1/2 cup pineapple chunks
- 1 tablespoon hemp seeds
- 1 tablespoon agave nectar

- 1 cup coconut water
- Ice cubes

Instructions:

1. Combine ripe avocado, spinach leaves, pineapple chunks, hemp seeds, agave nectar, and coconut water in a blender.
2. Blend until smooth and vibrant.
3. Add ice cubes and blend again for a refreshing chill.
4. Pour into a glass and enjoy this Avocado Green Goddess Smoothie.

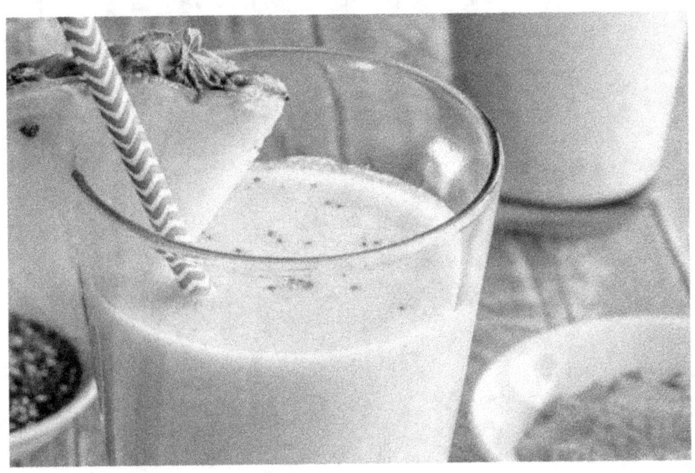

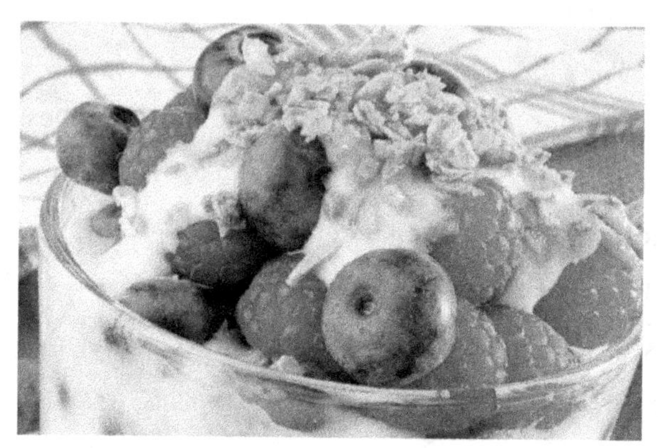

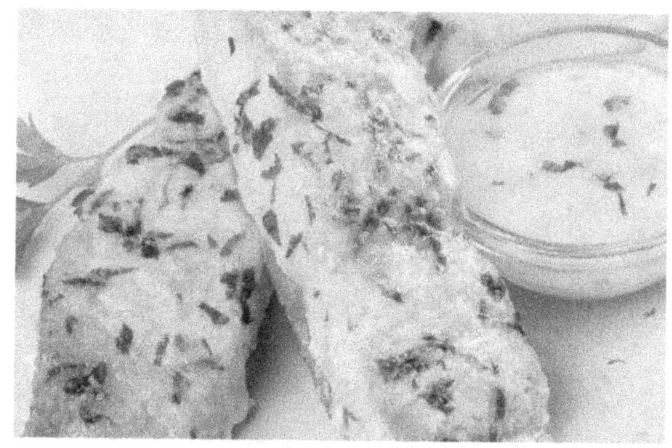

CONCLUSION

In conclusion, following a uterine fibroid diet may be a transforming experience for women seeking hormonal balance and uterine wellbeing. This detailed guide has offered useful insights into the role of diet in fibroid growth and control. By adopting smart food choices, women may empower themselves to flourish organically and enhance overall health.

The nutrient-dense meals in this book are not only tasty, but also specifically intended to promote hormonal balance and uterine health. These recipes, which include fibroid-fighting foods and emphasize key vitamins and minerals, provide a practical and pleasurable method to strengthen the body's resistance against fibroids.

It is important to understand the importance of living a healthy lifestyle in addition to making nutritional modifications. Regular exercise, stress management, and appropriate sleep complement nutritional efforts, resulting in a more comprehensive approach to uterine wellbeing.

This thorough book is intended to motivate women to take proactive measures toward hormonal balance and uterine health via mindful diet. By following a uterine fibroid diet and taking a holistic approach to health, women may empower themselves to flourish naturally and live full lives.

Happy Cooking!

MEAL PLAN

for a week

Week:...............................

	BREAKFAST	LUNCH	DINNER	SNACKS
MON				
TUE				
WED				
THU				
FRI				
SAT				
SUN				

Shopping list

_________________ _________________

_________________ _________________

_________________ _________________

Notes:

MEAL PLAN
for a week

Week:..............................

	BREAKFAST	LUNCH	DINNER	SNACKS
MON				
TUE				
WED				
THU				
FRI				
SAT				
SUN				

Shopping list

_______________ _______________

_______________ _______________

_______________ _______________

Notes:

MEAL PLAN

for a week

Week:...................................

	BREAKFAST	LUNCH	DINNER	SNACKS
MON				
TUE				
WED				
THU				
FRI				
SAT				
SUN				

Shopping list

Notes:

MEAL PLAN
for a week

Week:................................

	BREAKFAST	LUNCH	DINNER	SNACKS
MON				
TUE				
WED				
THU				
FRI				
SAT				
SUN				

Shopping list

Notes:

MEAL PLAN

for a week

Week:................................

	BREAKFAST	LUNCH	DINNER	SNACKS
MON				
TUE				
WED				
THU				
FRI				
SAT				
SUN				

Shopping list

Notes:

MEAL PLAN

for a week

Week:................................

	BREAKFAST	LUNCH	DINNER	SNACKS
MON				
TUE				
WED				
THU				
FRI				
SAT				
SUN				

Shopping list

Notes:

MEAL PLAN
for a week

Week:................................

	BREAKFAST	LUNCH	DINNER	SNACKS
MON				
TUE				
WED				
THU				
FRI				
SAT				
SUN				

Shopping list

Notes:

MEAL PLAN
for a week

Week:......................................

	BREAKFAST	LUNCH	DINNER	SNACKS
MON				
TUE				
WED				
THU				
FRI				
SAT				
SUN				

Shopping list

_______________   _______________

_______________   _______________

_______________   _______________

Notes:

MEAL PLAN

for a week

Week:...................................

	BREAKFAST	LUNCH	DINNER	SNACKS
MON				
TUE				
WED				
THU				
FRI				
SAT				
SUN				

Shopping list

___________ ___________

___________ ___________

___________ ___________

Notes:

MEAL PLAN
for a week

Week:................................

	BREAKFAST	LUNCH	DINNER	SNACKS
MON				
TUE				
WED				
THU				
FRI				
SAT				
SUN				

Shopping list

_______________ _______________

_______________ _______________

_______________ _______________

Notes: